Lektürehilfen
Arthur Miller
»Death of a Salesman«

Ernst Klett Verlag
Barron's Book Notes

Reihe: Lektürehilfen Englisch
Verfasser dieses Bandes: Liza McAlister Williams/Kent Paul

CIP-Kurztitelaufnahme der Deutschen Bibliothek

Williams, Liza McAlister:
Lektürehilfen Arthur Miller, »Death of a salesman«/
[Verf. dieses Bd.: Liza McAlister Williams; Kent Paul].
1. Aufl. – Stuttgart: Klett, 1987.
(Reihe Lektürehilfen Englisch) (Barron's book notes)
Einheitssacht.: Arthur Miller's Death of a salesman
ISBN 3-12-922228-6

NE: Paul, Kent:; HST
Vw.: MacAlister, Liza Williams → Williams, Liza McAlister

ISBN 3 - 12 - 922228 - 6

Ernst Klett Verlage GmbH u. Co. KG, Stuttgart 1987
1. Auflage 1987

Druck: Wilhelm Röck, Weinsberg
Einbandgestaltung: Hitz und Mahn, Stuttgart

CONTENTS

HOW TO USE THIS BOOK

You have to know how to approach literature in order to get the most out of it. This *Barron's Book Notes* volume follows a plan based on methods used by some of the best students to read a work of literature.

Begin with the guide's section on the author's life and times. As you read, try to form a clear picture of the author's personality, circumstances, and motives for writing the work. This background usually will make it easier for you to hear the author's tone of voice, and follow where the author is heading.

Then go over the rest of the introductory material—such sections as those on the plot, characters, setting, themes, and style of the work. Underline, or write down in your notebook, particular things to watch for, such as contrasts between characters and repeated literary devices. At this point, you may want to develop a system of symbols to use in marking your text as you read. (Of course, you should only mark up a book you own, not one that belongs to another person or a school.) Perhaps you will want to use a different letter for each character's name, a different number for each major theme of the book, a different color for each important symbol or literary device. Be prepared to mark up the pages of your book as you read. Put your marks in the margins so you can find them again easily.

Now comes the moment you've been waiting for—the time to start reading the work of literature. You may want to put aside your *Barron's Book Notes* volume until you've read the work all the way through. Or you may want to alternate, reading the *Book Notes* analysis of each section as soon as you have finished reading the corresponding part of the original. Before you move on, reread crucial passages you don't fully understand. (Don't take this guide's analysis for granted—make up your own mind as to what the work means.)

Once you've finished the whole work of literature, you may want to review it right away, so you can firm up your ideas about what it means. You may want to leaf through the book concentrating on passages you marked in reference to one character or one theme. This is also a good time to reread the *Book Notes* introductory material, which pulls together insights on specific topics.

When it comes time to prepare for a test or to write a paper, you'll already have formed ideas about the work. You'll be able to go back through it, refreshing your memory as to the author's exact words and perspective, so that you can support your opinions with evidence drawn straight from the work. Patterns will emerge, and ideas will fall into place; your essay question or term paper will almost write itself. Give yourself a dry run with one of the sample tests in the guide. These tests present both multiple-choice and essay questions. An accompanying section gives answers to the multiple-choice questions as well as suggestions for writing the essays. If you have to select a term paper topic, you may choose one from the list of suggestions in this book. This guide also provides you with a reading list, to help you when you start research for a term paper, and a selection of provocative comments by critics, to spark your thinking before you write.

THE AUTHOR AND HIS TIMES

Death of a Salesman opened on February 10, 1949, to reviews that acclaimed it a major new play. Within months Arthur Miller became world renowned as his play received the Pulitzer Prize, the New York Drama Critics' Circle Award, and the Antoinette Perry ("Tony") Award, among others. When Arthur Miller became famous, his grade school and high school teachers were puzzled. They couldn't remember him. Checking their records they found that as a student he had been most outstanding for his failures.

The issues with which Arthur Miller would later become preoccupied have clear beginnings in his family background. The second of three children of a middle-class Jewish couple, he was born in 1915 in New York City. His Austrian father was a manufacturer of women's coats, and his mother, the daughter of a manufacturer, had been a teacher. Miller knew from childhood the precarious hopes and disappointments of the business world, as well as its false dreams of extraordinary riches. This is the theme of *Death of a Salesman*.

It wasn't just his family background that influenced Miller. He grew up in the "roaring twenties," the decade we still think of as the giddiest in the history of our country. The world of business was prospering as never before. It was an age of distorted values—the pleasure of the moment, material richness, making money and showing it off. Miller's father hired more salesmen to sell his coats.

Miller played football and baseball, swam, skated,

and read adventure stories. "I passed through the public school system unscathed," he said later. While passing through, he failed many subjects, including algebra three times. You will recognize this athlete who doesn't apply himself in the character of Biff in *Death of a Salesman*.

When Miller was thirteen his family reached a crisis. Miller's father fell on hard times and had to move the family from Manhattan out to a small frame house in Brooklyn similar to the one in *Death of a Salesman*. Miller's sister recalls that he became "very handy with tools. He built the back porch on our house, and some of the roses he planted in the back yard are still blooming." Just as Arthur Miller loved working with his hands, Willy Loman loves to build things and tend a garden.

On graduation from high school Miller knew that his parents could not afford to send him to college. He wanted to go to the University of Michigan, but his grades were so poor that he could not qualify for admission. For a short while he worked for his father, but he couldn't stand the contemptuous way buyers treated his father and the salesmen. Self-respect became an important issue for him, as you'll see when you read *Death of a Salesman*. He got himself a job in a Manhattan auto parts warehouse. Miller was determined to make something of himself, and the fact that he achieved this goal gave him proof of any man's ability to perfect himself.

Meanwhile, he stumbled by chance on the Russian novel *The Brothers Karamazov*, which he had picked up thinking it was a detective story. (If you want to know what turned Arthur Miller into a playwright, read Dostoevsky's "great book of wonder" as he later called it. Have you ever been inspired by a book you read?) He read it on the long subway rides to work, and said later, "All at once [I] believed I was born to be a writer."

Miller saved nearly all of his fifteen-dollar-a-week salary, and after two and a half years he had enough for a year of college. He wrote the president of the University of Michigan an eloquent letter asking for one year to prove himself. He promised that if he did not do well, he would leave the university after his first year. The university accepted him in journalism, and he left the warehouse where he had built up the great affection for his co-workers documented in his play *A Memory of Two Mondays*. In the warehouse he had found a little community of people who cared about each other, in contrast to his father's business world. Among the questions always hovering over all his plays, including *Death of a Salesman*, are "Does anyone care?" and "How does a man make a home for himself in the world?"

At college Miller learned about a $500 award that was available for a play. He wrote one in six days, and won the prize. He felt he had begun what he had been born to do. At the University of Michigan he met many people who had strong political beliefs, ideas about how the world should be run. Listening to the debates heightened his concern about morality. Having won several more awards before graduating, Miller returned to New York in 1938 to write plays, but "in two months was on relief."

Odd jobs kept him going while he began to write for radio. Many of these jobs were manual labor, which gave him the background for his plays about working-class people.

In time, Miller wrote regularly for the best drama programs on radio. In spite of his impatience with radio's restrictions, he learned how to handle quick time shifts and how to blend reality and fantasy, a central strategy in *Death of a Salesman.*

Miller's first Broadway play was a failure, and he told himself that if the next one didn't succeed he would go into another line of work. In 1947 *All My Sons* put him on the map. Like *Death of a Salesman,* it deals with families and moral issues. While *Death of a Salesman* is about what society owes to individuals, *All My Sons* is about what individuals owe to society. It ran all that season and won many awards.

With the confidence of that success, Miller began *Death of a Salesman,* a more ambitious play. It immediately won extraordinary praise in this country, and also became one of the most frequently produced American plays abroad. A bestseller, unusual for a play, it has been read by millions of people who have never seen it.

Miller has been a public figure whose actions show what he stands for. During Joseph McCarthy's "witch-hunt" he refused to reveal the names of those at a meeting he had attended who might have been Communists. He was convicted of contempt of Congress in 1956, but two years later the Supreme Court reversed the conviction. He later actively campaigned for worldwide freedom of expression as an official of P.E.N., the international society of writers.

In addition to *Death of a Salesman,* Miller's plays include *The Crucible* (1953), *A Memory of Two Mondays* (1955), *A View from the Bridge* (one act, 1955; full length, 1957), *After the Fall* (1964), *Incident at Vichy* (1965), *The Price* (1968), and *American Clock* (1980).

Several of Miller's plays have been adapted into movies. In 1960 he wrote his first original screenplay, *The Misfits,* which starred his second wife, Marilyn

Monroe. Miller has also produced four books of reportage in collaboration with his third wife, the photographer Inge Morath: *In Russia, In the Country, Chinese Encounters,* and *Salesman in Beijing.*

The popularity of *Death of a Salesman* is timeless. Audiences around the world have been drawn to it, moved by its story of a longing for fulfillment. A notable revival was staged on Broadway in New York City in 1984.

THE PLAY

The Plot

Willy Loman, a traveling salesman, comes home in the middle of the night when he's supposed to be on a business trip. He tells Linda, his wife, that he couldn't keep his mind on driving, and kept going off the road because he was daydreaming. She urges him to ask his boss for a position with the company's headquarters in New York, so he won't have to travel anymore, and he agrees to see his boss the next day. He goes to the kitchen for a snack, and becomes involved in a memory of his son Biff. He has been talking to himself so loudly that he wakes Biff and his brother Happy, who are both there visiting, Biff from the West, and Happy from his own apartment in another part of town. The boys, now 32 and 34, talk over old times, worry about their father, and scheme about going into business together.

In the scene from Willy's memory, Biff, Happy, and Linda all suddenly appear on stage as they were fifteen years earlier, when the boys were teenagers. Biff, the favorite son, is the high school football captain. He is about to play an important game, and also about to flunk senior math, despite his friend Bernard's help studying. Bookish Bernard is not "well liked" by Biff's standards, and his father Charley, a salesman with his own business, is not "well liked" by Willy's standards. Still, for all his attempts to be "impressive," Willy is not doing well as a salesman, he confesses to Linda. Willy's thoughts shift further back in time to show him dallying with another woman in a hotel room.

Back in the present, Happy comes downstairs to calm his father, but is unsuccessful. The neighbor, Charley, comes in with the same intent, but Willy gets insulted when Charley offers him a job. Meanwhile, invisible to Charley, Willy's older brother Ben has arrived from the past. Willy is trying to have a conversation with two people at once, from different periods of his life, and ends up quarreling with Charley, who leaves. Now completely immersed in the past, Willy show off his teenaged boys to Ben, who invites him to move to Alaska. But Willy has convinced himself he has possibilities at home.

Returning to the present, Willy leaves the house to go for a walk. The family gathers to discuss his troubled situation. Linda says he is trying to kill himself because after 36 years with the company they have now taken away his salary and he is back on commission like a beginner, and broke because he can't sell anything. His pride is shattered and he's exhausted. Linda criticizes the boys for not respecting their father. Willy comes into the room, and the sons try to cheer him with their plan to open a sporting goods business. Biff will go to Bill Oliver, a former employer, and ask for $10,000 capital. Willy seems enthusiastic and gives advice about the interview. They all say goodnight with a feeling of hopefulness about the next day.

Act II begins the next morning. At breakfast, behaving like his old self, Willy tells Linda he will go into the city and ask for a job in the home office. She reminds him to get an advance because their last mortgage payment is due, and then they will own their home. Willy has put a lot of reconstruction into it and is proud of his carpentry skills. Linda tells him that the boys want to treat him to dinner at a restaurant.

At the office, Willy's young boss, Howard (son of

Willy's former boss) is playing a recording of his family on a new office machine. At last, when Willy can get a word in, he asks Howard for a New York position, but is refused even when he drops his request to forty dollars a week. Desperate, he raises his voice to Howard, who tells him to pull himself together and leaves the room. Shaken, Willy accidentally switches on the machine, which so unnerves him that he calls out to Howard to come and turn it off. Howard takes the opportunity to fire Willy, telling him to put away false pride and turn to his sons for support.

Ben reappears from the past, making a final offer to Willy of managing timberland in Alaska. It is Linda, loyal to Willy's unrealistic dream of success in business, who persuades him to turn it down. After Ben leaves, the family goes off to watch Biff play his big football game.

Back in the present again, Willy has somehow made his way to his neighbor Charley's office, where he has been coming every week for a loan so he can pretend to Linda he's making some money. Charley's son Bernard is there, now a lawyer on his way to Washington to try a case. Why did you turn out so well and Biff so poorly? Willy asks. Bernard answers that Biff could have gone to summer school to make up the math course, but instead he went to Boston to see Willy, and when he came back he had "given up his life." What happened in Boston? Bernard wants to know. But Willy becomes defensive about it, and Bernard leaves to catch his train. Charley comes in and gives Willy money. He again offers him a job but Willy refuses, though he does finally break down and admit he's just been fired. Willy dreamily comments that after all the years it's ironic that "you end up worth more dead than alive."

At the restaurant Happy has picked up a girl. Biff

arrives in a turmoil because Bill Oliver kept him waiting all day and never did recognize him. During the wait, and then when Oliver looked at him blankly, Biff had realized that for the last fifteen years he and his father and brother have been kidding themselves about who they are. Biff has stolen an expensive fountain pen from Oliver's office and run away. Now he is determined to tell Willy the truth, despite Willy's and Happy's attempts to alter the story. Sensing bad news, Willy slips into the past, and the boys witness him trying to answer all the voices in his head. Unable to cope with the past and the present at the same time, Willy goes into the washroom, and Biff, distraught, rushes from the restaurant followed by Happy with two girls he's picked up. Alone, Willy relives the scene in Boston fifteen years before when Biff discovered him in his hotel room with a woman. That was the moment when Biff decided his father was a "phony little fake."

Back in the present, when Biff and Happy finally get home, Linda brushes aside their feeble excuses about deserting their father and tells them to get out of the house and not come back. Willy is in the back yard planting seeds. He is having a conversation with Ben about a business proposition: cashing in his insurance policy by crashing his car and killing himself.

Biff comes outside to explain to Willy that since he can't seem to be around him without fighting, and he can't make of his life what Willy wants him to, he's going away. They argue. Biff shouts, "I'm not bringing home any prizes any more, and you're going to stop waiting for me to bring them home!" and breaks down in tears. Astonished, Willy realizes that Biff loves him after all, because he "cried to me." Everyone goes to bed except Willy, who, somehow cleansed and absolved by Biff's love, roars off in his car to make the final profit—selling his life—that he is convinced will get Biff on his feet financially. The family and neighbors gather and get ready to go to the funeral.

In the Requiem, the family is at the cemetery. They talk about why Willy died. Biff says, "He had the wrong dreams." Charley replies, "A salesman [has] got to dream, boy. It comes with the territory." and Happy adds, "It's the only dream you can have—to come out number-one man." Linda has the last word: "I can't understand it, Willy. I made the last payment on the house today. . . . And there'll be nobody home. We're free and clear," she sobs. "We're free. . . ."

The Characters

Willy

Willy Loman is a traveling salesman in his sixties. We know from the title that he is going to die. He is experiencing an emotional crisis. His past, recurring to him in vivid scenes, is interfering with the present. Each time he returns from an episode in the past, he brings with him a discovered piece of information that throws new light on his troubled present. He's realizing that he's lived his whole life by the false standard that you can lie and cheat to make your fortune as long as you are "well liked." Arthur Miller wrote, "if I could make him remember enough he would kill himself." What does Willy have to remember? Why does Willy have to remember it now?

Willy's name—Loman—is significant: it suggests "low man" on the totem pole. The company Willy has worked for all his life has recently stopped his salary and is paying him only commissions on sales, like a beginner. They claim he's not getting the business, and they can't afford to keep him on. Now he's having trouble driving—he can't pay attention so the car keeps going off the road. If he can't drive, traveling (the only kind of selling he knows) will have to stop.

He'd like to be able to count on his two sons, but he knows he can't. The older one, Biff, disappears for months at a time between jobs in the West. Willy idolizes him, but for years whenever they have been together they quarrel. Happy, the younger son, has a steady job but is taking bribes and wasting his money. Willy's wife Linda is his mainstay, but he's reduced to supporting her with handouts from a neighbor.

Now Willy is recalling the most important events in

his life—his life is passing before his eyes—as he searches to understand what went wrong. Miller has called the play a "confession."

What Willy wanted in life was to make a lot of money by being well liked. As he relives past experiences, we see that he went after what he wanted with energy and ingenuity. But he wanted success so badly that he lost a realistic sense of himself. He forgot that he loved making things with his hands, and he ignored standards of fair play.

Willy is like a boy in his impulsive enthusiasm and sudden discouragement. The many contradictions in his character reveal a man who doesn't know himself at all. For instance, he will borrow money from his neighbor Charley but refuses to take a job working for him. He'd rather die than work for a man he sees as inferior.

Until the day he dies Willy never stops dreaming up ways to better his life. He is full of imagination, even to the point of committing suicide in a scheme to make $20,000 on his insurance policy. Because of his eternal hopefulness and resourcefulness, he is a lovable character who gives an actor great scope.

Willy's struggle was long and finally tragic. Linda says, "A small man can be just as exhausted as a great man." Miller writes, ". . . this man is actually a very brave spirit who cannot settle for half but must pursue his dream of himself to the end." We can find joy in what Willy manages to learn about himself—and in the forgiveness and love he wins from his favorite son.

Linda

"You're my foundation and my support," Willy tells Linda. Even then he may be understating her devotion to him. She is the model of a loving, devoted, patient wife. When she married Willy, his dreams must have seemed like all she ever wanted in life.

Those dreams have turned into a lifetime of frustrations. Disappointed and worried, Willy sometimes treats Linda cruelly or insensitively, but she understands the pain and fear behind his behavior, and forgives him those moments. Miller tells us, "she more than loves him, she admires him." A man with as fragile a sense of self-worth as Willy cannot tolerate his wife's disagreeing with him, so Linda has long practiced ignoring her own opinions. She has always supported Willy in his illusions about himself—he had so convinced her of his possibilities at home that she talked him out of his one chance to go to Alaska with Ben. She manages to be cheerful most of the time.

Linda as she was in the past is the way Willy chooses to remember her (as is the case with all the characters when he recalls them). Willy's guilt turns her into an even sweeter and more noble woman, a shining example of a "good woman." We also see that it is Linda who has kept a clear picture of their finances. When Willy boasts of big sales, she gently questions until she learns the truth—never rebuking him for exaggeration (lying). She does the best she can with their meager income to pay their endless bills. She must manage well, for we learn in the Requiem that she has made the final payment on their house and they're "free and clear."

Linda has made a child of her husband, always indulgent and affectionate with him. She senses that Willy is in trouble, and to protect him she is terrifyingly tough on the two grown-up boys. She is a good and understanding mother, but will not tolerate her sons crossing their father. After the boys abandon their father in a restaurant for dates with women they've picked up, she blisteringly attacks both of them: "There's no stranger you'd do that to!"

Linda knows her beloved Willy is a "little man," but she feels he deserves at least the respect of his sons: "Attention, attention must finally be paid to such a person." Probably Linda speaks the playwright's attitude toward Willy more than any other character in the play.

Biff

Biff is 34 and has just come home again from farm work in the West. A star athlete in high school, Biff would conquer the world, thought Willy. Biff's success would mean that Willy had raised him right. But Biff is not a success. He feels "mixed up," confused, uncertain, as though he's wasting his life.

Is he wasting his life, though? When he talks about the farms where he's worked, from the Dakotas to Texas, he speaks with such enthusiasm and eloquence that his brother calls him a "poet." That he doesn't make enough money to "get ahead" makes him feel that he isn't fulfilling his father's expectations. He has been forced to move from job to job because he steals. Now he has come home to try to figure out how to get into something permanent—a job or a marriage. But at home he fights with his father.

While he was growing up, Biff had idolized his father, and Willy had thought Biff could do no wrong. But during Biff's senior year of high school something happened between him and Willy that no one else knows anything about. The two of them have not admitted, even to each other, what happened, but it has affected their relationship ever since. Biff's return upsets Willy, and brings back the first experience from the past.

Of course, the Biff we see in the past is Willy's romanticized version, but still we may begin to see how his problems developed. Willy favored Biff so clearly over his younger brother, Happy, that Hap would literally jump up and down trying to get attention. All Biff's friends fawn over him, eager to do whatever little job he'll give them. Bernard, the neighbor's unathletic son, loves and admires Biff and helps him with his studies.

Willy believes—and makes Biff believe—that anyone so confident, so gorgeous, so natural a leader has the right to make his own rules. He doesn't punish Biff for "borrowing" a football from school; he lets Biff drive without a license; he encourages Biff to steal from a nearby construction site. Biff so believes in his father that when he fails a math exam, he's certain Willy can talk to the teacher, and goes to Boston to find him. When Biff discovers something about his father that shocks him, he gives up on himself and on his father. He refuses to grow up and accept responsibilities. At 34, Biff says to his brother, "I'm like a boy."

Biff is the inheritor of the same false ideals that are killing his father. Like his grandfather and father before him, Biff is good with his hands and has an appealing personality, but he doesn't want to start at the bottom. He says to Willy, "You blew me so full of hot air I could never stand taking orders from anybody."

Biff, like his father, has refused to see what he has actually done with his life. But on this return to his parents' home a crucial difference between Biff and Willy develops. Biff is aware of his own unhappiness. He takes a long and clear-eyed look at himself—and at his father. He insists on telling his father what he sees: that he has never been what his father thinks he is. From that new and painful truth, Biff is able to understand Willy and to forgive him and to give him the love that has long been stifled between them. The hope we are given at the end of the play is that Biff is capable of accepting himself. This balances the futility of Willy's life.

Biff says Willy had the wrong dreams, "All, all wrong." What becomes of Biff after his father's death is an intriguing question, but he'll do it on his own terms. He has become his own man.

Happy

Happy is 32, two years younger than Biff. Like his brother, Happy is an attractive and powerful man. The playwright comments that sexuality lingers on him like "a scent that many women have discovered." Hap's name suggests happy-go-lucky. He seems to have inherited his mother's good nature and acceptance of the way things are.

In the scenes from the past we see Happy doing everything within his power to get his father to notice him. He keeps up a vigorous routine of exercises, and his refrain as a boy is to ask his father whether he's noticed that he's losing weight. It's almost as though he's asking Willy whether he sees him at all.

In the present Hap has found a similar line. "I'm gonna get married, Mom. I wanted to tell you," he throws in at inappropriate times, desperate for attention. He's learned how to say what people want to hear, but neither of his parents takes him seriously. Linda says, "Go to sleep, dear," and Willy offers, "Keep up the good work."

On the face of it, the grown-up Happy appears to have achieved the things Willy wanted for his boys—a steady job, the social life of a popular single man, a car, and his own expensive apartment. However,

Happy turns out to be a sham. Instead of a buyer, he is an "assistant to the assistant" buyer. He takes bribes from salesmen who want to do business with the company he works for. He seduces women in whom he has no real interest, especially women engaged to executives above him in the corporate structure. He confesses to his brother that he has "an overdeveloped sense of competition." He is lonely and longs for the chance to prove himself. He wants to meet a woman of substance like his mother. But he never will. He is a man without scruples and has no real desire to develop a life with values. He is generous enough to send his father to Florida for a vacation, but he isn't interested in spending time with him. By the end of the play it is clear that he is callous toward both his parents.

Hap abandons his father in the moments Willy is most distraught, saying to the girls he's picked up, "No, that's not my father. He's just a guy." It's no wonder Happy rejects his father after his father's lifetime rejection of him. But over his father's grave he exclaims, ". . . Willy Loman did not die in vain. He had a good dream. It's the only dream you can have—to come out number-one man." Happy seems fated to be another Willy.

Charley

Charley is a large, unimpressive man about Willy's age. He is Willy's neighbor and the father of Biff's schoolmate Bernard. Unconcerned about appearances, Charley first appears in pajamas and robe, when he comes over in the middle of the night to see why Willy's home.

Making clear that his play is not an attack on business in general, Miller writes that "the most decent man in *Death of a Salesman* is . . . Charley whose aims are not different from Willy Loman's. The great difference between them is that Charley is not a fanatic. Equally, however, he has learned how to live without that frenzy, that ecstasy of spirit which Willy chases to the end."

Charley stands in contradiction to everything Willy believes in. He is not concerned about being well liked, and says to Willy: "Why must everybody like you? Who liked J. P. Morgan? Was he impressive? In a Turkish bath he'd look like a butcher. But with his pockets on he was very well liked." Willy recalls Charley in the past, looking ridiculous in knickers his wife bought for him. Charley doesn't care about sports in the least. He has no ability with tools. His relationship with his son Bernard has been casual, and he has never given him advice. Charley isn't obsessed about the business world.

However, Charley is successful in business. To make money is as natural for him as carpentry is for Willy. Charley is prospering well enough that he can regularly lend Willy money which, although Willy assures him he's keeping strict accounts, Charley knows he'll never see again.

Charley is not threatened by Willy's abilities, which are different from his. He admires the ceiling, telling Willy that "to put up a ceiling is a mystery to me." He is stern about Willy's low standards of fair play, and impatient with his childlike dreams, urging Willy all through the years to "grow up." Charley is a realist. He knows that Willy doesn't much like or respect him, but that doesn't keep him from caring about Willy and seeing his good qualities. Despite Willy's rejection of his offers, Charley twice tells him that he could use him in his firm. In the final hours when he is reviewing his life, Willy recognizes what Charley has meant to him, and as he leaves Charley's office, stops to say with real feeling, "Charley, you're the only friend I got."

Bernard

Bernard initially comes into the play in an episode Willy is imagining, and Willy exaggerates what the young Bernard was like. A bookworm, spending little time outdoors, he is several times mockingly called "an anemic" by Willy and his boys. Both Bernard's behavior and the Lomans' making fun of him provide much of the humor in the first act. Later, in the present, Willy wonders how such a pathetic excuse for a kid could become the self-possessed lawyer of the present.

Even in the first-act caricature, however, we note the qualities that will permit Bernard to build a career. He works hard at his studies. As much as he admires Biff, he can't go along with his friend's stealing and cheating. But he never turns his back on Biff when they're students, and tries to help him with his schoolwork.

In the present Bernard has developed a promising career, has a wife and two sons, and keeps a friendly relationship with his father in which both are self-sufficient. He hasn't forgotten how promising Biff was, though, and we feel that he still honestly wishes Biff well. He tries to tell Willy that he would help Biff by leaving him alone.

Uncle Ben

Ben, Willy's older brother, whom he scarcely knew, is completely an imagined figure in the play. Willy tells Charley that he recently learned that Ben has died, so we know when Ben walks into the scene with Charley that he is an apparition Willy has summoned in his anguished search to understand his life.

From the moment we see Ben he turns out to be a highly idealized figure, for Willy's memory turns him into a god. Willy says about him, "There was the only man I ever met who knew the answers." Ben is an imposing-looking man dressed in sophisticated clothes and projecting great authority. He is fearless and ruthless and enjoys his success enormously, constantly chuckling over it. He has an air of always thinking about secret and important things. He fathered seven sons.

For Willy, Ben is a "man who had all the luck." Even his mistakes become profitable. Ben tells about how he left to find their father in Alaska when Willy was three or four. However, "I had a very faulty view of geography, William. I discovered after a few days that I was heading due south, so instead of Alaska, I ended up in Africa. . . . [W]hen I was seventeen I walked into the jungle, and when I was twenty-one I walked out. And by God I was rich."

So Ben personifies ideal success, the realization of the wildest dreams a man might have. In his quest to make some sense of his failed life, Ben serves Willy as a guide—an older brother's role—who appears to him every time Willy is most desperate. Ben is the inspiration for the fierce daring Willy sees in committing suicide. Ben encourages him toward this action that will put Willy in control of his life, and allow him to beat the world that beat him.

Howard

Howard Wagner is thirty-six and inherited the company from his father. It is extremely difficult for Howard to face up to firing Willy. Whenever Willy tries to bring up business, Howard diverts the conversation with talk about his family. We learn that he is a devoted father and that he is fascinated by gadgets, always taking up the newest fad. Howard is not an insensitive man, but Willy for a long time has not been pulling his weight. We feel that he is somewhat sorry for Willy, but his responsibility is to running a profitable company.

The Woman in Boston

The Woman in Boston exists only in the past, as Ben does. She works at one of the companies to which Willy sells. She is a dignified, middle-aged, single woman who likes Willy because he makes her laugh. She is lonely, just as Willy is when he's on the road, and their affair is casual. It's painful for her that she cannot expect anything enduring from the relationship, and looking for some reward, she prizes highly the silk stockings Willy gives her. In the first act Willy is trying to persuade her to stay overnight; in the second act, when Biff discovers them, she is obviously spending the night with Willy. She is embarrassed and humiliated, and in the transitory nature of her relationship with Willy she feels like a "football," as she tells Biff in leaving.

Miss Forsythe and Letta

Miss Forsythe and Letta are the women Happy picks up in the restaurant while he and Biff are waiting for Willy. In some commentaries these two characters are described as prostitutes, but they're not. They're young women looking for a good time that evening in the same spirit Happy and Biff are.

Stanley

Stanley is the young waiter in the restaurant. Early in the sequence we see the joking attentiveness that is the way to better tips. However, Stanley has a compassion worth noting. After Happy and Biff have left their father in the washroom, Stanley is concerned about Willy and helps him to his feet. In gratitude Willy tips him, and Stanley slips the bills back into Willy's coat pocket.

Jenny

Jenny is Charley's secretary, who has to handle Willy's erratic behavior on his visits to borrow money from Charley. She is relieved when Bernard takes responsibility for Willy while Willy is waiting for Charley.

Other Elements

SETTING

When the lights come up, the first thing we see on stage is the suggestion of a small frame house. The front wall is open, and the stage directions say that "an air of the dream clings to the place." The set is designed to minimize the boundaries between past and present. The same areas used conventionally for scenes in the present are also used for scenes in the past as free spaces where characters can step "through the walls." Only a few key objects tell us what each room is; for example, a refrigerator, a table, and three chairs represent the kitchen. In Willy and Linda's bedroom is a brass bedstead, a straight chair, and a silver athletic trophy that symbolizes the peak achievement of Biff's life. Upstairs is the boys' old bedroom, with two small beds.

In front of the house is an empty area that "serves as the back yard as well as the locale of all Willy's imaginings and of his city scenes."

Behind the roof the outlines of apartment buildings tower threateningly over the little house, which seems as fragile as Willy's dreams. The stage directions call the house "a dream rising out of reality," and this reflects the central theme of Willy's longing to fulfill himself in a world where making money is the only acceptable goal.

The stage directions say the play takes place "today." Its premiere was in 1949. Nowadays, some productions of the play leave the time of the action unspecified, and for others the program reads "1949." While the emotions of the play will never be outdated, the authentic details on every page place it in 1949. The brand names of the household appliances, Biff's football game at Ebbets Field (a baseball stadium where the Dodgers played, long gone from Brooklyn), the price of dinner in the restaurant ($1 for a specially prepared lobster)—all are details of life in the United States shortly after World War II.

A key detail that dates the play is the memory Willy describes of driving in his car with the front windshield open. In some early cars the windshield could be opened on a nice day for a breezy drive. At the time of the main action of the play, it had been many years since cars had windshields that could be opened, and so Willy is alarmed when he realizes he thought he was back in the era when he was a young salesman.

THEMES

1. WHAT'S HAPPENED TO THE AMERICAN DREAM?

Historically the American dream meant a promise of freedom and opportunity for all. A new frontier lay open and anyone who worked hard could expect to have a happy and prosperous life. Today, however, we think of the American Dream in a less idealistic way, as the instant business success of those who are ruthless or lucky. The critic Harold Clurman wrote, "Instead of the ideals of hard work and courage, we have salesmanship . . . a certain element of fraud—the accumulation of profit being an unquestioned end in itself."

We Americans seem to feel we deserve money and material things as our birthright. Advertising reinforces our desire for possessions, often making us want things we either don't need or can't afford. Then when we don't have enough money to buy everything we want, we feel cheated somehow.

Willy Loman is a perfect example of someone who feels betrayed because he can't achieve the financial goals society has conditioned him to strive for. He worships the goddess of success, but he doesn't have the talent or the temperament to be a salesman, his chosen career. When he fails as a salesman, no other measure of success—the love of his family, his talent as a carpenter, and so on—can comfort him. He believes that a person who fails in business has no right to live.

Biff opposes his father's attitude. He chooses to be poor, if necessary, and to do the things he loves, rather than sacrifice his freedom in the mad pursuit of money. This disagreement between father and son provides the central dramatic tension of the play.

Happy wants business success and follows in his father's unhappy footsteps to try to get it. The neighbor, Charley, is content with modest wealth. His son Bernard chooses a different path, achieving professional and financial success in law, a field to which he's tempermentally and intellectually well-suited. All these characters have chosen their own ways of responding to the American Dream.

It's important to remember as you read the play that it's not a criticism of salesmanship itself, but of the pursuit of money as an end in itself.

2. LYING, EXAGGERATING, REVISING

Because he doesn't want to face his failure, for years Willy has been lying to himself and to others, fantasizing and fooling himself into a false vision of his own popularity. This erroneous view of himself, or "false pride," as his boss calls it, gets in the way of Willy's relationships.

3. IDENTITY

"Who am I?" is a question we all ask. Willy, whose father and older brother went away when he was very young, has always felt insecure about how he should be conducting his life. Most of the time he covers up his feeling "kinda temporary" about himself with boasts of "hot air" (as Biff calls it). Only when he's deeply in trouble does he ask advice—"what's the secret?"—from Ben, from Charley, from Bernard, all of whom have achieved the financial success he longs for. If Willy could have accepted and made the most of his good qualities, he might not have struggled all his life to fit into the wrong mold. Note that Willy forced this mold not only onto himself but also onto his sons, causing them the same confusion over identity.

4. UNREALISTIC EXPECTATIONS

All during the course of the play, Biff is trying to come to terms with, and ultimately rid himself of, his father's dreams and expectations. Willy expects him to be great in business because he was great in sports. Believing that Biff has all the makings of a success, Willy sees his son's failure to amount to much as a deliberate act of "spite." In turn, Biff feels his father is "mocking" him.

5. NATURE VERSUS THE CITY

Willy's father was a wanderer, a pioneer, a maker of flutes, and a musician. Willy's older brother Ben was an adventurer who lived in Africa where he got rich on diamond mines and invested in Alaskan timberland. Willy's sons were strong and skillful athletes in high school. All of these people, including Willy himself, have an affinity for the outdoors, for physical skills, for a happy-go-lucky, carefree existence.

Early in his career as a salesman Willy would drive through the beautiful countryside with the front windshield of his car open. He would come home to his garden and the little house he was fixing up, and play with his sons. But soon the city closed in on them, tall apartment buildings blocking the light from reaching the garden. At the same time Willy's financial demands closed in on him, overpowering him with the necessity for making money. Biff says that men like them should be doing carpentry work out in the country. In spite of Willy's objection that "even your grandfather was better than a carpenter" (note the value judgment), the expression of Willy's true nature is the flute, "telling of grass and trees and the horizon," as the stage directions say.

6. MORTALITY VERSUS IMMORTALITY

All creatures must die; most leave nothing behind them. It is human to fear this mortality and to wish that instead of vanishing anonymously we could leave a monument of our work and suffering. Arthur Miller wrote of the "need to leave a thumbprint" as being as strong a need as hunger or thirst. Willy wants to make an impression, to be remembered after his death, to "give something" to Biff, and his inability to do any of these haunts him. His life has been futile: he is old, poor, scorned by his peers and his sons. His final attempt to make a legacy for Biff is his suicide, which he feels will earn the $20,000 of his insurance policy.

7. SUICIDE

The question of why Willy commits suicide is of course central. The title *Death of a Salesman* raises it even before the play begins. Though you will form your own opinions of the forces that drove Willy to kill himself, here are some reasons to consider as you read: escape, from the empty and bitter reality of his life; revenge, for his sons' disrespect and resentment; power, in taking action when everything seems hopeless; courage, to lay down his life; victory, finally being able to make a profitable deal, and, by redeeming his life insurance policy, giving his son a fortune;

understanding, that he went wrong, but at the last minute knowing that his son loves him anyway.

8. A TRAGIC HERO

Critics have hotly debated the questions of whether Willy is a tragic hero or whether *Death of a Salesman* is a tragedy. Dramatic tragedy was invented and defined by the Greeks. Aristotle said a play has to have four elements to qualify as a tragedy: 1) noble or impressive characters; 2) the main character's discovery or recognition of a truth about himself; 3) poetic language; and 4) the ability to arouse and then soothe the audience's pity and fear. Some critics consider that *Death of a Salesman* is debatable on all four elements, while others think the play meets all these criteria. Arthur Miller argued that times have changed—we no longer live in an era dominated by kings and queens—and so maybe our definition of tragedy should change, too. (See the section of this guide on Influences for more on this subject.)

Though he is a common man—Low-man—Willy was later described by the author who created him as "a very brave spirit who cannot settle for half but must pursue his dream of himself to the end." Though Willy did not have great intellectual powers, Miller claims he did have a self-awareness—otherwise he would not have killed himself when he realized his life was meaningless.

The difference between Willy and his salesman neighbor Charley is that Willy is intense and passionate and cares about his dream enough to sacrifice his life to it. A tragic hero is someone with the dedication to die for a belief, but also someone who has a tragic flaw or limitation that defines him as a character and makes the tragedy happen. He has alternatives, but he chooses to live in a certain way that brings about his downfall. All of this is true of Willy.

tragic

LANGUAGE

Miller has an infallible ear for natural dialogue. To Miller a person's background matters, so he makes his characters speak in a true-to-life style, or vernacular. Their language reflects all the directness, humor, and pain of working-class people. Listen to Biff: "I'm mixed up very bad. Maybe I oughta get married. Maybe I oughta get stuck into something." This is matter-of-fact vocabulary, full of bad grammar, slang, and casual, sloppy pronunciation. Yet Biff is instinctively going right to the heart of his confusion.

A play usually shows its characters at the peak of some change or crisis, and *Death of a Salesman* does this to the fullest measure. A family that has never been very direct or honest, in trouble financially and emotionally, is suddenly thrown together after several years, and the things they say to each other are explosive and full of meaning. Because this family has always fooled itself with lies and exaggerations, readers must be alert to contradictions, to people not saying what they mean. The pauses, too, seem significant, and the things they don't say.

At moments the characters seem almost poetic in the intensity of their emotions. In the special circumstances of disaster they are moved to phrase their thoughts more formally than they otherwise might, as when Charley, standing at Willy's grave, says, "Nobody dast blame this man."

The times when characters are most agitated are when they use metaphors, or poetic comparisons. For example, in Act I, when Linda is accusing Biff of shiftlessness, she says, "A man is not a bird, to come and go with the springtime." In Act II, when she is begging Biff on the phone to help his father, she says, "Be loving to him. Because he's only a little boat looking for a harbor." A few pages later when Willy is desperately demanding a New York job from Howard, he says, "You can't eat the orange and throw the peel away—a man is not a piece of fruit!" In times of emotional intensity, a metaphor is often the most graphic or vivid way to illustrate a point.

Arthur Miller's skill in blending ordinary and poetic speech is one of the reasons this play is a modern classic. It touches a universal nerve of realism and poignancy. Indeed, a great many people wrote to Miller that their own lives had been revealed in the play.

POINT OF VIEW AND FORM

Death of a Salesman is not a strictly realistic play. It recognizes that the world of dreams is as real as the waking world: one's imagination is as real as the actual events of one's life. Unlike most plays, this one tries to capture both of these realities and present them with equal vividness on the stage.

Because the scenes from the past are actually recurring in Willy's mind as he conducts his present life, they are not strictly flashbacks—a term we have consistently avoided in this guide. Compare the flashbacks in a movie, where only the audience, not the characters, are viewing scenes from before the start of the story. What makes this play different is that the journeys into the past are Willy's clinical symptoms, his repressed experiences surging back into memory. As they unfold in his mind, they affect how he views events in the present.

In his daily life Willy has recently been moving uncontrollably from the present to the past and back again, much to the distress of himself and his family. As we read the play we must keep in mind that all time is in the present, as these memories of Willy's crowd in. We need to watch for clues that signal these transitions.

For Willy a word or a thought in conversation brings back a related incident from the past in all its original intensity. Therefore, we follow Willy from scene to scene as different times and places flow into each other. The theatrical set remains the same because, as Miller wrote, "the mere fact that a man forgets where he is does not mean that he has really moved."

Arthur Miller set out in *Death of a Salesman* to paint a true portrait of how one person thinks, and, in fact, his original title for the play was *The Inside of His Head*. Miller wanted to show us the feelings, observations, and associations that occur daily in our "subjective process of thought-connection," as he later put it. He was striving for a believable and accurate pattern of thought and language, with all its confusions and contradictions. In the "Introduction to the *Collected Plays*," Miller wrote, "I was convinced only that if I could make him remember enough he would kill himself, and the structure of the play was determined by what was needed to draw up his memories like a mass of tangled roots without end or beginning."

INFLUENCES

When Arthur Miller began reading plays in college, Greek tragedies made a profound impression on him. He says that he was drawn to the Greeks "for their magnificent form, the symmetry." While he claims he barely understood the characters or comprehended the stories, he recognized the classic construction. "That form has never left me; I suppose it just got burned in."

As soon as *Death of a Salesman* opened, critics began writing about its relation to Greek tragedy, usually pointing out that Willy doesn't qualify as a tragic hero.

Without mentioning his critics, Miller replied with an essay titled "Tragedy and the Common Man." *Death of a Salesman* does have a shattering emotional impact that corresponds to that of a Greek tragedy. There are some other similarities—the inevitable movement toward death of the protagonist (or central character) with growing self-awareness, the single story without subplots, the unity of time (*Death of a Salesman* takes place within the course of about twenty-four hours)—but they are of limited significance.

More important for an understanding of the form of *Death of a Salesman* is a familiarity with German expressionism. Expressionism sought to depict the inner life of characters. It went further than realism or naturalism, which traced the lineal development of a story through external details of environment. Expressionism used symbols to evoke the unseen and the unconscious, and so expressionist plays were "cool" in their approach: objective, stylized, impersonal.

Miller took the form and made it "warm" and humane. He later wrote that *Death of a Salesman* "desired the audience to forget it was in a theater even as it broke the bounds, I believe, of a long convention of realism. Its expressionistic elements were consciously used as such, but since the approach to Willy Loman's characterization was consistently and rigorously subjective, the audience would not ever be aware—if I could help it—that they were witnessing the use of a technique which until then created only coldness, objectivity, and a highly stylized sort of play."

The incidents from the past that Willy recalls in the present are an "expression," or dramatization, of what's going on inside Willy's mind. An observer in the present would simply see Willy talking, mumbling to himself. Our witnessing those recollected episodes lets us experience Willy's process of thought.

The Story

ACT I

Willy Loman, a traveling salesman, returns home unexpectedly to his little house in Brooklyn one night. As he appears, we hear a flute, "small and fine, telling of grass and trees and the horizon."

NOTE: Observe the surprising presence of a flute, an instrument often associated with nature and the woods, in this urban setting. We'll see the growing significance of this instrument.

Willy carries his sample cases into the kitchen, sighing as he puts them down. He is exhausted. Not expecting him home, his wife Linda is worried and calls out to him. Willy attempts to reassure her, but as he enters the bedroom the flute fades and he says, "I'm tired to the death." He had driven only a short distance on his way to New England when he began to daydream and had trouble keeping the car on the road, so he had to turn back. Linda urges him to ask for a spot in the company's headquarters in New York. He says he will.

Their two grown sons are asleep in their old room upstairs. Biff, the older one, returned that morning from working on a farm in the West. He has been working at seasonal farm jobs—this one for $28 a week, which at age 34 feels humiliating—for many years. Father and son had had a fight when Willy asked Biff if he was making any money. Willy is still upset about the fight, though Linda, the peacemaker, takes Biff's side, saying he has to "find himself."

"Not finding yourself at the age of thirty-four is a disgrace!" Willy explodes.

NOTE: The tension between father and favorite son is evident: dollars and cents mean less to the son than to the father. This clash in values is classic, isn't it?

"Biff is a lazy bum!" Willy complains, but he betrays contradictory feelings a moment later when he says, "In the greatest country in the world a young man with such—personal attractiveness, gets lost. And such a hard worker. There's one thing about Biff—he's not lazy." This contradiction seems funny to us (the author intended it to get a laugh) but in addition we have learned in the first few lines of the play that there is a conflict between Biff and Willy, and also within Willy himself. We have already seen that Willy is full of exhaustion and disappointment, and that's not what he had expected from life. As a young person you have a dream of how your life will be when you grow up. Willy's was to be a highly successful businessman. But his time is now running out, he has failed to reach his goal, and he wants his son to fulfill his dreams. He loves his son, and he tries to make him into something he's not.

Willy recalls the time when there were elm trees and a garden in the back yard. Now he feels boxed in by new adjacent apartment houses, and longs for space and natural surroundings.

NOTE: Willy seems to feel choked by urban life as it takes over the neighborhood. Nature symbolizes freedom for him, and the expression of his natural self and his longings. Remember the sound of the flute was "telling of grass and trees" when it introduced Willy; the flute will return throughout the play at the times Willy comes closest to his true nature. We'll see the image of trees again later, too, for example when Willy says in a crisis, "The woods are burning, boys!" Willy's life has gotten far away from the things that he is good at, like working with his hands or planting a garden. The time is gone when all his dreams were seeds waiting to flower.

Linda promises a drive in the country on Sunday with the windshield open. Willy corrects her, saying that the windshield doesn't open on the new car. When she protests that he just said he was driving with it open, he realizes that all day he has been imagining a car he had nearly twenty years before. It becomes clear to us—and to Willy—that he is increasingly lost in the past. It must be terrible for him not to be able to tell past from present. Shaken, Willy goes down to the kitchen to get something to eat.

Upstairs Biff and Happy have been awakened by their parents' voices. Happy is staying over at home after taking Biff on a date. Both are immediately worried, because lately they have been noticing Willy's strange behavior. Imagine how it would feel to have your father start talking to himself. You would be nervous and embarrassed. Biff tries to find excuses for their father's bad driving, but Happy, who has driven with him, says Willy just doesn't pay attention.

> *Happy:* . . . He stops at a green light and then it turns red and he goes. *He laughs.*
> *Biff:* Maybe he's color-blind.
> *Happy:* Pop? Why he's got the finest eye for color in the business. You know that.

Willy has trained his sons well—in the end everything relates to business. Even personal characteristics are valued in terms of their usefulness.

Happy has been looking for the chance to talk to

Biff about their father. But Biff is still mad about that quarrel this morning, and asks, "Why does Dad mock me all the time?" Happy points out that when Willy is mumbling to himself he usually seems to be talking to Biff. Perhaps if Biff had a regular job, Happy hints, their father would stop worrying. Bristling at the suggestion that he is entirely responsible, Biff shifts some of the blame to Happy.

NOTE: We all recognize the conflict between brothers who have grown up to be quite different. Biff cares about saving his soul, Happy about making money. Happy is more like Willy, but isn't it ironic that Willy likes Biff better?

Still, Biff does admit that he himself is worried about his inability to settle down. For six or seven years after high school he tried various jobs in business, but he hated the routine, the competition, the having to "get ahead of the next fella." He fled the business world to the outdoor work he loved. "Go West, young man" was a very real call to him. In the wide open spaces he felt free. (Remember, nature also means a great deal to Willy.)

Though Biff loved working outside, he has made little money at it, which doesn't fulfill the expectations he's inherited from his father. He says,

> . . . There's nothing more inspiring or—beautiful than the sight of a mare and a new colt. And it's cool there now, see? Texas is cool now, and it's spring. And whenever spring comes to where I am, I suddenly get the feeling, my God, I'm not gettin' anywhere! What the hell am I doing, playing around with horses, twenty-eight dollars a week! I'm thirty-four years old, I oughta be makin'

> my future. That's when I come running home. And now, I get here, and I don't know what to do with myself.

NOTE: Look at the dialogue throughout the play. People usually talk in short, simple sentences so that a long speech like this one is unusual.

Hearing this passionate outburst, Happy calls Biff a "poet" and an "idealist." No, says Biff, "I'm like a boy." But he is no longer a boy, good at sports, the apple of his father's eye; now he's a man, but with none of the confidence of an adult. He is full of uncertainty, resentment, and guilt over "wasting" his life.

NOTE: Biff's dilemma is interesting. Is his problem simply that he refuses to grow up? His parents accuse him of this. That's an easy accusation, but sometimes such behavior comes from a refusal to compromise one's ideals. In order to grow up you have to have a role model, but Biff doesn't want to become like his father.

Biff asks if Happy is content in his job. We see that on the surface he looks happy and successful, but he really isn't. "It's what I always wanted," Happy says, but confesses that he's lonely and stifled. He has lots of girlfriends but nobody he cares about. He has a car and his own apartment but he hates taking orders from "petty" people, including his boss. He's in good physical shape, and sometimes he wants to strip down in the middle of the store and start boxing with the merchandise manager to show him his real merit. What does this say about him? Maybe he hasn't outgrown his adolescent preoccupation with athletic prowess.

Hearing Hap's complaints, Biff has an idea: "Why don't you come out West with me?" They dream of buying a ranch, "us[ing] our muscles." Together they could be happy, not care about the rest of the world. They feel the old bond of their childhood again. It's an appealing idea to escape to a dream world where the two of them could have fun just like the old days. But is it practical?

It is Happy who suddenly asks, "The only thing is—what can you make out there?" Who cares, counters Biff, if you have peace of mind? Here is the essence of the difference between the brothers. Happy is caught in the system: "I gotta show some of those pompous, self-important executives over there that Hap Loman can make the grade." With pride he boasts about the gorgeous girls he takes out. He confesses that his latest conquest is engaged to one of the executives in the store—a pattern he's been getting into. He "ruins" them and then goes to their weddings. "Maybe I just have an overdeveloped sense of competition or something."

NOTE: Notice how Happy uses the word "competition." Competition is what drives Willy onward, and what Biff is trying to escape from. It tempts Happy to seduce women he doesn't want, to take bribes to get business, and then to justify himself with phrases like, ". . . everybody around me is so false that I'm constantly lowering my ideals." Here is a restatement of one of the themes of the play: the betrayal of ideals.

When Happy can't achieve his goal of being a big shot at work, he feels cheated. The American dream is out of his reach so he himself resorts to cheating.

Biff has an idea how he could get some money to buy a ranch. In high school he had worked for a businessman named Bill Oliver. When he quit, Biff remembers, Oliver said, "If you ever need anything, come to me." Now he decides to ask Oliver to lend him $10,000 to get started out West.

Like many incidents in this play, this first mention of Oliver gives a different version than later references. Our impression of Biff's relationship with Oliver changes within a few lines when Biff says, "I wonder if Oliver still thinks I stole that carton of basketballs." This is a revealing question. He probably did steal them, but has always denied it, even to himself. All the Lomans have a remarkable ability to revise events in a light favorable to themselves.

Biff and Happy's middle of the night chat is interrupted by Willy talking loudly in the kitchen. He is reliving a scene from the past in which Biff is waxing ("Simonizing") the car. Hearing this, Biff, who is already upset, gets angry. Happy pleads with him not to leave home again, and to have a heart-to-heart talk with their father, but Biff can only express disgust that Willy would shout aloud his memories with no regard for their mother. What self-respecting person would allow himself to lose control like this? Biff doesn't realize that Willy is at his wits' end. As he gets into bed, Biff says to himself, "That selfish, stupid . . ."

NOTE: By the time the light has faded on their bedroom, stage lights have gradually come up on Willy downstairs in the kitchen. Light and music are our key signals for scenes changing. In this instance the orange silhouettes of the apartment houses are fading above the roof, symbolizing the fading away of the present and Willy's troubles. Though Willy is eating a snack, his mind is far away, in the past. A light effect suggesting sun shining through the leaves of overhanging trees fills the stage, turning it into an outdoor area—the backyard. This leaf pattern always announces the scenes of Willy in the past at home. The sound of the flute reinforces the feeling of warmth and hopefulness associated with the past.

At first we hear only one side of the conversation. Willy is imagining his boys polishing the family car. He tells them to use newspaper on the windows, chamois cloth on the hubcaps. Biff is polishing the car so carefully because he has a date, so we assume he's about sixteen, just old enough to drive. We hear Willy cautioning him not to waste his time on girls, but to pay attention to schoolwork. We see Willy at first smiling at an empty kitchen chair, but gradually he begins to look through the wall of the kitchen. His focus shifts to the area outside the house. Willy says that as soon as the boys have finished waxing the car, he has a surprise for them.

Offstage we hear Biff's voice: "Whatta ya got, Dad?" But Willy won't tell them until they've finished the car, saying, "Never leave a job till you're finished—remember that." (Knowing what we know about Willy's unhappiness in his job in the present, this line has a ring of painful double meaning for us.)

At this point a remarkable thing happens on stage. Biff and Happy, who only moments before were in bed upstairs, appear from the side of the stage dressed as teenagers, apparently fresh from waxing the car.

NOTE: In the original 1949 production, and in later ones, great care was taken to make this transformation as magical as possible. Special beds with trapdoors or elevators were invented so that as soon as their conversation upstairs ended and the lights went down in their room, the actors, without being seen, could get offstage and change their costumes as Willy began talking. When the same actors walk into Willy's scene as teenagers, we are taken completely by surprise, and we can't understand how the trick was done. The effect of this staging device is to make us realize how abrupt are the shifts in Willy's mind between the present and the past. The appearance of Biff and Happy as they looked in the past gives these recalled scenes as much reality to us, the audience, as they have for Willy.

The stage directions tell us that Happy is carrying a pail of water and Biff is wearing an athletic sweater and carrying a football. Willy gives them the surprise, a punching bag he brought home with him on his return from a selling trip. The boys are ecstatic, especially when they see that it has a famous pro's signature on it. Happy, who is two years younger than Biff and anxious to please both him and their father, is hopping around; he is the kid brother, always trying to get his share of attention. He lies on his back now and pedals his feet in the air, showing how he's training to get in shape. Sports and competition—that key word again—are central in this family.

Biff shows off his new football. When Willy asks where he got it, Biff evades the question by saying the coach told him to practice his passing. "That so? And he gave you the ball, heh?" says Willy. With a laugh of guilt mixed with pride, Biff confesses that he "borrowed" it from the locker room. Laughing with him, Willy tells him to return it. We see that his attitude toward the theft, though he says Biff was wrong to do it, is a little bit indulgent and conspiratorial. Biff is his favorite son who can do no wrong.

Happy, jealous of the attention Biff is getting, says to Biff, "I told you he wouldn't like it!" But Willy defends him, saying, "He's gotta practice with a regulation ball, doesn't he? Coach'll probably congratulate you on your initiative!" This is the kind of justification Willy is good at: twisting something bad into something good.

Willy begins telling the boys stories of his selling trip to New England. He says he had coffee with the mayor of Providence and "sold a nice bill" in Waterbury. He boasts about how popular he is: "They know me, boys, they know me up and down New England. The finest people." He promises to take them up there this summer.

He brags that someday he'll have his own sales business, like their neighbor, "Uncle" Charley—but bigger and better than his, "Because Charley is not—liked. He's liked, but he's not—well liked." This is a recurring idea; we must remember it. It is Willy's way of measuring success: "well liked" enough to make your fortune by it.

We learn that Biff has been made captain of the football team and that he'll be playing in a big game on Saturday. Taking Willy's hand he says, ". . . just for you, I'm going to break through for a touchdown." Biff ignores Happy's protest that he's supposed to pass, not make points. But when we hear that, we realize that Biff is planning to use the game to his own advantage, that like his father he makes up his own rules to suit his needs.

Charley's son, Bernard, a studious, scrawny boy,

comes on stage, whining that Biff is supposed to be studying with him today. Their class will take the Regents exam next week, and the results will determine who gets college scholarships. When Happy starts boxing with Bernard, Bernard fights back with the information that he overheard their math teacher threatening to flunk Biff. Willy angrily reminds Bernard that with sports scholarships offered by three universities, the high school wouldn't dare flunk him. "Don't be a pest, Bernard!" says Willy, and adds to his boys, "What an anemic!"

All the Lomans are in the habit of making fun of Bernard. He lacks the flashiness, the rugged physique, and the "gift for gab"—the qualities of ideal manliness according to Willy. "Bernard is not well liked, is he?" Willy asks after he's gone. Biff answers, "He's liked, but he's not well liked." We recognize that line from Willy's description of Bernard's father, Charley.

Willy insists on thinking of himself and his sons, especially Biff, as "well liked," and therefore successful because they can make people do anything for them. Ironically, we will soon see that studious Bernard and hard-working Charley are the ones who achieve real success in the end, not only because they are smart, but because unlike Willy they know where their strengths lie.

It's so important to Willy to see himself as well liked that he fills his sons full of pictures—lies, really of his popularity. His wife Linda, however, isn't as easily fooled. She arrives onstage carrying a basket of washing, and when the boys go off to hang it up for her, she greets Willy warmly and asks, "Did you sell anything?" Willy names a large figure. She excitedly takes a pencil and paper from her apron pocket to figure his commission. At that, he backs down and tells her the true figure. They calculate how much money they owe: monthly payments on the refrigerator, washing machine, vacuum cleaner, new roof, and so on. When he has to face the bills, we learn how contradictory Willy's thinking really is:

Willy: A hundred and twenty dollars! My God, if business don't pick up I don't know what I'm gonna do!
Linda: Well, next week you'll do better.
Willy: Oh, I'll knock 'em dead next week. I'll go to Hartford. I'm very well liked in Hartford. You know, the trouble is, Linda, people don't seem to take to me.

Willy tells her that people seem to laugh at him or not notice him, that he talks too much, and that he's too fat. She's never before heard him speak this way. We are witnessing a private and painful moment, a crisis of self-doubt and self-recognition. Linda, however, loves him as he is, not as he wishes to be. She tells him that to her he's the handsomest man in the world.

The scene is about to change. Through Linda's words we hear a woman laughing from the darkness at the side of the stage. The signals of music and lighting draw our attention away from Linda. As Willy is saying how lonely he gets for her on the road, and how worried he is about not being able to make a living, he walks across the stage toward a woman who is just finishing getting dressed.

The bridge between the scenes is Willy's unfinished line, "There's so much I want to make for—" The woman picks up the words and changes the meaning. "Me? You didn't make me, Willy. I picked you." They are in Willy's hotel room in Boston, and Willy doesn't want her to leave. She is about his age, "proper looking," works in one of the stores he visits. It's clear they're having an affair. She thanks him for the silk stockings he's given her. She promises to see him again next time he's in town because he's a kidder and makes her laugh. She's laughing as they kiss and say goodnight. Her laughter as she leaves blends with Linda's laughter, returning us to the scene of Linda and Willy's conversation. Stage lights come up in the kitchen.

Linda is darning a pair of silk stockings, and still talking about how handsome he is. In a frenzy of guilt about the other woman Willy angrily tells Linda to throw out the stockings. Everything starts caving in on him. His memories are clamoring in his brain. Bernard runs in, shouting that Biff has to study and he's driving the car without a license. Linda chimes in that Biff shouldn't have taken the football and he's too rough with the girls. The other woman is laughing in the background. To all of them he yells "Shut up!" but they continue finding fault with Biff until Willy explodes, "There's nothing the matter with him!" Linda leaves the kitchen almost in tears. Alone, Willy seems to wilt in defeat. All the warm light of the scenes from the past is gone. When we notice the apartment buildings towering over the house again, we know we are back in the present.

Happy comes downstairs to try to calm Willy. He promises to give his father enough money to retire. Willy scornfully reminds him he makes $70 a week and wastes most of it on women. "Where are you guys, where are you? The woods are burning! I can't drive a car!"

We see that this is the final disaster for Willy. As a traveling salesman his life depends on being able to drive. But today he nearly hit a child on the side of the road, and was so scared he had to turn back. Why hadn't he gone to Alaska, years ago, with his brother Ben?

Charley arrives from next door in his bathrobe. He has heard the noise and wonders what's the matter, but Willy takes his presence as an insult. Sending Happy to bed, Charley takes out a deck of cards and offers to play a game of casino. As they play, he casually mentions that he wants to take a trip and could use Willy's help in his business. It's not the first time he's offered Willy a job, and as usual Willy takes offense. He refuses to admit defeat in front of Charley, whom he views as a man with no personality. "I got a good job," Willy lies. He seems to resent Charley out of all proportion.

Suddenly a new character enters Willy's imagination: his older brother Ben, dapper with an umbrella and suitcase. Willy speaks to Ben, and hearing the name, Charley asks, "Did you call me Ben?" Willy makes the excuse that Charley reminds him of Ben, whom they learned had died recently. For a few minutes things get very mixed up as Willy tries to listen to both Ben in his mind and Charley in the room at the same time. Charley finally asks several times in frustration, "What're you talkin' about?" To cover up his own odd behavior and because he feels on the defensive, Willy accuses Charley of cheating in the card game. Charley slams the door in a huff, leaving Willy free to enter completely into the new scene with Ben.

Ben has come to invite Willy to make a new start in Alaska. Willy was only three when his brother left home to seek his fortune and ended up in Africa with investments in diamond mines. He hasn't seen Ben since. Now Ben is here for a few minutes before catching a train for Alaska.

> **NOTE:** All the hopes of a lifetime seem to Willy to be wrapped up in his successful brother. Ben is a stranger but Willy has made him into a hero. Having no one to advise him, Willy relies on his imagined concept of Ben to encourage him when he feels insecure. We see Ben as he looks through Willy's eyes: worldly, fabulously rich, sure of what he wants and how to get it. He is a kind of puppet or cartoon of Willy's dreams, not a fully developed character in the play. The same is true of Linda as a young woman and of the high school–aged boys. They exist in the imagined scenes only as Willy perceives them to be.

Young Linda has come in, and the teen-age boys. They gather around Ben as he tells about his father, a wanderer whom Willy barely remembers. He played the flute, Ben says, and sold the flutes he made from town to town. He was "a very great and a very wild-hearted man"—a true salesman. (We see now why it is so appropriate for the music that represents something pure in Willy to be flute music.)

Willy boasts that he's bringing up the boys to be "rugged, well liked, all-around." Ben invites Biff to box with him, then trips him, saying, "Never fight fair with a stranger, boy. You'll never get out of the jungle that way." (Is this an honorable motto? Do we agree with it? Willy seems to. Stealing or lying seem to be acceptable in his code, if he can twist them around to suit his cause.) Eager to show Ben how handy his boys are, he sends them running to the nearby construction site of an apartment building to steal some sand to make a new front step.

Charley comes over, looking youthful and rather silly in a pair of knickers. He warns that the watchman at the building will call the cops if the boys don't stop stealing materials. Willy justifies their thefts:

Willy: I gave them hell, understand. But I got a couple of fearless characters there.
Charley: Willy, the jails are full of fearless characters.
Ben: *(clapping Willy on the back, with a laugh at Charley)* And the stock exchange, friend!

We can view Charley's and Ben's reactions as the two battling sides of Willy's conscience.

The next few minutes are a whirlwind. Bernard runs in saying the watchman's chasing Biff. Linda is upset by Ben's sudden visit. Charley is upset about sales in his business being so bad. Willy is in a panic at the prospect of Ben leaving so soon, and in a tumble of words he confesses that although he has "a fine position here" (a lie), he stills feels "kind of temporary about myself." How should he bring up his boys, he cries out. Willy hangs on every word as Ben, leaving, assures him he's doing a first-rate job. The highest authority in Willy's world has spoken, and it's enough for Willy. "I was right! I was right! I was right!" he shouts until Linda, in her nightgown and robe of the present, hurries in to find him.

Linda tries to soothe him, but he's shaken by the emotion of his memory. He shuffles off in his bedroom slippers to take a walk, unable to cope with the sudden shift back to the present.

Biff and Happy come downstairs. For the first time they all talk honestly about Willy.

Happy: I never heard him so loud, Mom.

Linda: Well, come around more often; you'll hear him.

Biff: Why didn't you ever write me about this, Mom?

Linda: How would I write to you? For over three months you had no address.

Linda explains that Willy is worse when Biff is around, perhaps because he can't open up to him. She gently accuses Biff of not having "any feeling" for his father. Pay respect to your father, she says, or don't come home anymore.

The sound of Willy offstage calling his name from deep in one of his memories infuriates Biff. He tells his mother to stop making excuses for Willy, who often treated her badly through the years. Happy starts to object, but Biff cuts him off saying, "He's got no character." Linda defends him. "He's not the finest character that ever lived. But he's a human being, and a terrible thing is happening to him. So attention must be paid."

What is the terrible thing that is happening to Willy? Is it just that he is losing his bearings? Or is it that he is becoming so tormented by his confusions and failures that he can no longer face his life?

We learn from Linda that Willy has just lost his salary, after 36 years with the company. For five weeks now he has been on a straight commission, like a beginner. When Biff and Happy express indignation, Linda cuts them short: "Are they any worse than his sons?" She claims that the boys were glad to see their father when he was supporting them, making money, but now, like the company, they have no use for him. His old contacts are dead or retired; he drives 700 miles each way and doesn't make a cent—so no wonder he talks to himself! He borrows $50 a week from their neighbor Charley (now we understand why Willy resents Charley so much) and pretends to Linda that he earned the money.

"How long can that go on?" Linda asks. At 63 years old he has worked all his life to make ends meet for children "he loved better than his life" who no longer appreciate him. He's exhausted: "a small man can be just as exhausted as a great man," she asserts.

NOTE: This line is possibly one of the most important in the play, and Arthur Miller defended this idea in his essay "Tragedy and the Common Man." Previous definitions of tragic drama claimed that only heroes having "rank or nobility of character" were worthy of having plays written about them. But today, unlike in ancient Greek or Shakespearean times, kings and queens are less relevant to us. Miller claims that the "underlying fear of being displaced . . . from our chosen image of what and who we are in this world . . . is as strong, and perhaps stronger, than it ever was." Miller believes that all of us can identify with the struggles of a modern character: ". . . the tragic feeling is evoked when we are in the presence of a character who is ready to lay down his life, if need be, to secure one thing—his sense of personal dignity."

Linda is holding nothing back now. She calls Happy "a philandering bum" and asks Biff "What happened to the love you had for him?" But now it's Biff's turn to lay some cards on the table. He reminds his mother that Willy threw him out of the house. She has never understood why, but Biff will say darkly only, "Because I know he's a fake and he doesn't like anybody around who knows!" Angrily Biff adds that he'll stay in this city, which he hates, and give his father half his salary. What more do you want?

What Linda says next brings the boys to shocked attention. "He's dying, Biff." She has heard from the car insurance inspector that a series of "accidents" in the last year were really Willy's attempts to kill himself. A witness had seen him deliberately drive off a small bridge. And then Linda has found a rubber tube in the basement and a new valve on the gas pipe—apparatus that would allow Willy to asphyxiate himself by breathing gas. She has not had the nerve to confront Willy about these things; she feels it would be an insult to his pride. But every day she fears for his life.

NOTE: Why doesn't she confront her husband with the evidence? Doesn't she want to save him from this terrible action? Of course she does. But Willy is a strong character. To discuss suicide with him would be to discuss failure, and that is what Willy can't face. We must keep in mind something else: Linda, too, hates to admit that Willy is not all he longs to be. She's as committed to the fantasy of success as he is. We'll see that at the moment when he might have gone to Alaska with Ben, Linda urged Willy to think of his "good position" at home.

Feeling guilty, Biff promises to make a new start in business, even though he feels he's not cut out for it. He will try once again to be what Willy wants him to be. Just try to please people, advises his brother, especially the people you work for.

The thought of flattering superiors is too much for Biff. He exclaims, "They've laughed at Dad for years, and you know why? Because we don't belong in this nuthouse of a city! We should be mixing cement on some open plain, or—or carpenters."

Willy comes in. The boys now see him with new eyes, knowing that he is considering suicide. They watch him nervously, and treat him with kid gloves. Scornfully Willy says, "Even your grandfather [the flute player] was better than a carpenter. You never grew up."

Willy has overheard more than that. "And who in the business world thinks I'm crazy?" We hold our breath: how will Willy respond to this bold statement of his failure? No one in this family speaks honestly until he's absolutely forced to, and here is Willy stumbling onto Biff's true feelings.

But Willy's ego, the lie he unfailingly carries with him, bounces back. Go to any department store in Boston, he sneers to Biff. "Call out the name Willy Loman and see what happens! Big shot!"

Biff is teetering between fear of upsetting his father and anger at the "fake." When Willy asks him why he's always insulting him, Biff's at the boiling point. It has become clear to him that he can't be around his father without fighting, so he'd better just go away forever. He tells his father he's leaving early tomorrow.

But Happy has another idea in mind, and without consulting Biff he adds, "He's going to see Bill Oliver, Pop." All of a sudden Biff is in an awkward position. That wasn't what he meant about "leaving." Should he say so? Or should he make a supreme effort after all, and try to do what would please his father?

He decides on the second choice. He wants Oliver to set him up in a sporting goods business, he says. His father asks how much Oliver will give him, but he says he hasn't even gone to see him yet.

Willy: Ah, you're counting your chickens again.
Biff: Oh, Jesus, I'm going to sleep!
Willy: Don't curse in this house!
Biff: Since when did you get so clean?

NOTE: Biff is hinting at something. Remember when he told his mother Willy is a fake? Biff is harboring some kind of secret about his father, and it is poisoning his entire relationship with him. When you find out something upsetting about a person whom you love, especially a parent, it's hard to treat him the same way afterward. Willy is not far wrong to say Biff is always insulting him.

To break up the impending fight, Happy interrupts with another idea. Excitedly he describes it: he and Biff will sell a line of sporting goods, the Loman Line. They will form two teams and have sports competitions to advertize the goods. It wouldn't be like business; instead it would re-create the old family closeness and utilize their athletic skills.

We realize that Happy is using Biff's own tactics: a sales pitch for teaming up together. It works. Biff is enthusiastic. And Willy is ecstatic. He starts giving Biff advice on how to make the best of the interview with Bill Oliver: dress conservatively, talk as little as possible, don't make jokes. Is this the same Willy Loman talking? He is really warming to the picture of the interview. "Start off with a couple of your good stories to lighten things up. It's not what you say, it's how you say it—because personality always wins the day." Willy's true philosophy goes against even his own best advice.

As they are building this fantasy, we can see Linda brightening with renewed hope that maybe things will be all right after all. But each time she adds a word of encouragement, Willy cruelly tells her to stop interrupting. Finally Biff can't stand it anymore, to see his father, whom he doesn't respect, abusing his mother, who humbly takes it. When at last he bursts out, "Stop yelling at her!" Willy suddenly goes quiet, looking beaten and guilty, and leaves the room.

Begging him to say goodnight nicely to his father, saying "It takes so little to make him happy," Linda hurries out after Willy. As the boys start talking again about the Oliver scheme, they get excited and go up to Willy. They say an awkward goodnight, Willy repeating his grandiose advice: "If anything falls off the desk while you're talking to him . . . don't pick it up. They have office boys for that."

As Biff leaves the room, Willy is recalling the great football game at Ebbets Field when Biff in his gold uniform led his team to the city championship. A Hercules, Willy calls him.

Might this be the time, Linda wonders, to ask something that has been on her mind since her talk with Biff? "Willy dear, what has he got against you?" But he brushes her aside. "I'm so tired. Don't talk any more." Do you think he knows what she is referring to? Or is he really too tired to focus?

We see Biff go to the gas heater, which is now glowing behind the kitchen with blue light. He takes the piece of rubber tubing Willy has hidden behind it. With a look of horror on his face, he goes upstairs to his room.

ACT II

In the morning Biff and Happy are up and gone before Willy wakes. He's slept well for the first time in months. He's in a hopeful mood brought on by the boys' plan to start a business. He'll plant a garden, he tells Linda eagerly, and someday move to the country, raise vegetables and build guest houses for each of the boys to stay in when they visit with their families. (If only he could admit that building and gardening are what he's best at and should have been doing all his life.)

He's going to ask his boss for a New York job. While he's at it, Linda reminds him, ask for an advance of $200 to cover recent bills. Willy complains that just as he gets something like the refrigerator paid for, it wears out.

NOTE: Willy is caught in a trap we are all familiar with: built-in obsolescence. We are consumers of "essentials" like modern appliances, autos, even houses. Because they are expensive, we pay for them in monthly installments that can stretch out over years. Often by the time they are paid for they are so old they have to be replaced, and the cycle starts again. This is a torment to Willy, whose tiny income is gobbled up each month by the family bills. No wonder Linda is frugal, and darns her stockings. And no wonder every time he sees her doing it, Willy is seized with guilt over having had a mistress, to whom he gave new silk stockings.

It is an important day for several reasons. First, Willy and Linda know that this month's mortgage payment will be the last, and that finally, after 25 years, the house will belong to them. Wrapped up in the house are years of memories—Biff was nine when they moved in—and hours of Willy's own labor remodeling and repairing it.

Second, Willy is confident that he can convince his boss to keep him in the New York office. His positive attitude is catching, and both he and Linda feel exultant:

Willy: I will never get behind a wheel the rest of my life!
Linda: It's changing, Willy, I can feel it changing!
Willy: Beyond a question.

The third cause for excitement is that the boys have invited their father to dinner at a restaurant that evening. Flattered, Willy hurries off to catch the subway into the city to see his boss.

The phone rings. Biff has called to make sure Linda told Willy about their dinner date. She can hardly wait to confide a discovery to him: the rubber hose is gone from behind the water heater. Of course when she learns Biff took it, she's disappointed, but still she feels happy because Willy was "in such high spirits, it was like the old days!" She reminds Biff to make an extra effort to be nice to his father tonight, "Because he's only a little boat looking for a harbor." The metaphor is appropriate: Willy has been exhausted and tossed about by troubles, and his rescue seems to have something to do with Biff. Linda is so sensitive to the importance of Biff's love and respect for Willy that she instinctively puts it in the strongest words she knows: "Biff, you'll save his life." She is not exaggerating, the way most of us do when we use that phrase.

A new scene is set on the other side of the stage as Linda hangs up the phone. Howard Wagner, Willy's young boss, comes out pushing a portable table, the kind used for typewriters. On it is a wire-recording machine, an early version of the tape recorder. As the stage lights fade on Linda and come up on Howard, we can see Willy trying to get Howard's attention.

Howard is playing with his brand new recorder, an

invention that in 1949 is not yet widespread in offices. He took it home the night before and recorded himself, his wife, his young son and daughter, and now he is excitedly playing back the recording as Willy tries to get a word in. Each time Willy tries to speak, Howard hushes him, listening to the machine. Finally Howard turns it off, saying he's going to throw out "my camera, and my bandsaw, and all my hobbies" in favor of having fun with this machine.

We are getting a picture of Howard as a successful man with plenty of money, a model family, and the free time to tinker with one expensive gadget after another—you probably know people like that, who take up and drop each fad as it comes along. Willy tries to be enthusiastic about the wire-recorder.

> *Willy:* I think I'll get one myself.
>
> *Howard:* Sure, they're only a hundred and a half. You can't do without it. Supposing you wanna hear Jack Benny, see? But you can't be home at that hour. So you tell the maid to turn the radio on when Jack Benny comes on, and this automatically goes on with the radio. . .

Willy doesn't admit to Howard that he doesn't have a maid (and perhaps not even a radio), and that $150 is about the amount of his monthly bills he is struggling so hard to meet. But he plays along with the lie: "I'm definitely going to get one. Because lots of time I'm on the road, and I think to myself, what I must be missing on the radio!" Surprised, Howard asks, "Don't you have a radio in the car?" Caught in his own lie, Willy fumbles, "Well, yeah, but who ever thinks of turning it on?"

Suddenly Howard realizes that Willy is supposed to be in Boston. "What're you doing here?" he asks. This is Willy's big moment. Bravely he announces, "I've come to the decision that I'd rather not travel any more." He asks Howard for a spot here in New York, and a $65-a-week salary. Each time Howard tries to interrupt, Willy keeps on talking, finally saying, "Speaking frankly and between the two of us, y'know—I'm just a little tired."

There isn't a place for him in the New York store, Howard says. Most of the company's business is sales to other stores by traveling salesmen, and "you're a road man, Willy." Willy is desperate and won't take no for an answer. He's been with the firm since Howard's father was a young man and Howard himself was a newborn baby, Willy reminds him. Howard is looking for his lighter, and Willy hands it to him—just the kind of gesture he advised his son Biff to avoid during his interview. When Howard maintains there's no opening for him here, Willy drops his price to $50.

"But where am I going to put you, kid?" Notice that a man half his age is calling Willy by the derogatory term, "kid," which shows how little respect Howard has for the older man. Willy asks him point-blank if he thinks he can't do his job:

> *Willy:* Look, it isn't a question of whether I can sell merchandise, is it?
> *Howard:* No, but it's a business, kid, and everybody's gotta pull his own weight.

What Howard is really saying is yes, you don't do a good job.

Willy is getting angry, and he uses his final ammunition, the thing that means most to him: the story of his life. He tells of wanting to go to Alaska, but being inspired instead by an old and well-respected salesman called Dave Singleman, who could pick up the phone and do his business without stirring from his hotel. When he died—"the death of a salesman" in the smoking car on the train to Boston—his funeral was attended by hundreds of his business associates. Willy winds up his plea passionately with what amounts to his philosophy of life: "In those days there was personality in it, Howard. There was respect, and comradeship, and gratitude in it. Today, it's all cut and dried, and there's no chance for bringing friendship to bear—or personality. You see what I mean? They don't know me any more."

Restless and uninterested—or perhaps embarrassed—Howard has not looked at Willy during his story, but now he picks up on Willy's last line about not being known by the buyers anymore. "That's just the thing, Willy," he starts, but Willy is not to be distracted from what he wants. He lowers his bid to $40, but still Howard says no. At this, Willy again brings up Howard's father, but even the mention of this authority figure seems to have no effect on Howard, who starts to leave, saying he has to see some people.

Willy has become panic-stricken as he sees his last chance slipping away. His voice rising, he stops Howard: "I'm talking about your father! There were promises made across this desk! You mustn't tell me you've got people to see—I put thirty-four years into this firm, Howard, and now I can't pay my insurance! You can't eat the orange and throw the peel away—a man is not a piece of fruit!"

Willy tries to tell him that in 1928 he averaged $170 a week, but Howard doesn't believe him, tells him to pull himself together, and leaves. Stunned, Willy realizes he's been yelling at his boss. He leans on the desk, the same desk Howard's father, Frank, used to occupy. As he speaks in his imagination to Frank, he accidentally bumps into the wire-recorder. A childish voice starts repeating the state capitals in alphabetical order. The babble of the wire-recorder parallels the babble in Willy's mind. He calls out frantically to Howard, who rushes back in and unplugs the machine. Willy's composure has cracked; he presses his hands to his eyes and says he needs a cup of coffee. He feels defeated, and his only aim now is to maintain his dignity and get out of the room. He'll keep traveling, he concedes; he'll go to Boston. But Howard has something to say:

Howard: I don't want you to represent us. I've been meaning to tell you for a long time now.
Willy: Howard, are you firing me?
Howard: I think you need a good long rest, Willy.

Howard tells Willy to come back "when you feel better" and maybe they can "work something out." But they both know that will never happen and that Willy is being fired for good. Willy protests that he has to earn money. Ask your sons to help you out, suggests Howard: "This is no time for false pride." But of course Howard has hit on one of the major characteristics of Willy's personality. To tell Willy not to have false pride is like telling him to stop breathing.

His sons are busy on a "very big deal" says Willy, and anyway he can't impose on them like a "cripple." Let me go to Boston, he begs, grasping Howard's arm. With effort Howard keeps his temper, ordering Willy to get hold of himself and then go home.

Alone for a moment Willy stares exhausted into space. Music is heard. Ben comes in and Willy relives a scene from the past, when Ben was on his way back from Alaska. He has bought timberland, needs someone to manage it, and offers Willy the job. Linda as her younger self comes in. She doesn't like Ben, she thinks he's ignored them all these years only to appear suddenly and stir up trouble. Last time he praised the boys for fighting and stealing, and unsettled Willy with talk of making a fortune in the wilderness. Now here he is back again, trying to lure them away from their life here.

What does Linda fear they will lose by going? She has swallowed Willy's golden lie of the promise of success and happiness. Willy has been having a good year and his boss, Frank Wagner, has said he'll be a partner in the firm someday if he keeps up the good work. He's "well liked," and doing well enough to be happy right here, right now, Linda insists. She has taken Willy's optimistic fantasies so to heart that she defends them against even him.

Willy is bouncing back and forth between Ben's and Linda's reasoning, two sides of his own mind. I'm building something here, he tells Ben, who simply replies, "What are you building? . . . Where is it?"

Ben is leaving to board his ship back home to Africa. In an effort to keep him a moment longer, Willy shows off Biff, who is about to go and play his big football game at Ebbets Field. Three universities want to give him scholarships. "It's who you know and the smile on your face" that get you places in life, according to Willy. You can make your fortune from the contacts you develop.

Willy feels insecure enough about this philosophy to want a final encouragement from his older brother whom he probably will never see again. "Ben, am I right?" he asks. "I value your advice." Ben says only that he could get rich in Alaska, and leaves. For the rest of his life Willy will be tortured by the idea he was wrong not to go to Alaska.

Charley's boy, Bernard, runs in. When he sees the Lomans he is relieved that they haven't left for the game without him. Happy has the honor of carrying Biff's helmet, and Bernard settles for carrying the shoulder pads, which will entitle both of them to accompany Biff into the locker room. Willy hands out pennants and gives Biff a fatherly pep talk, and Biff replies, "I got it, Pop. And remember, pal, when I take off my helmet, that touchdown is for you." There is a strong bond of closeness between them. They are both taking the competition of this day very seriously.

As they are all about to leave for Ebbets Field, Charley saunters in. Knowing how much the football game means to Willy, he teasingly asks him where he's going, a baseball game? Enraged by his jokes, Willy retorts, after the others have gone, "I don't think that was funny, Charley. This is the greatest day of his life." But Charley merely asks him when he's going to grow up. He can't see getting so worked up about sports, and that's one big difference between the two men. Willy is now so angry he's ready to fight—"Put up your hands!"—probably partly because he has always been jealous of Charley, who seems to succeed without doing any of the things Willy feels are important: sports, working with tools, impressing people with stories of a lot of money.

Of course Charley doesn't fight, he just walks away laughing. Willy follows him, shouting names at him. We now notice the two signals that the scene is changing: lights coming up on a different area of the stage, and music, in this case rising to a "mocking frenzy" to indicate Willy's anger and disorientation.

Offstage Willy is still shouting as the lights come up on Bernard, now a grown man. He's sitting in his father's office as Willy's voice gets louder and nearer. Charley's secretary, Jenny, asks Bernard to go out in the hall and quiet Willy down, but before he can get up Willy comes in. He jokes coarsely with Jenny and is shocked to realize who the self-assured young man is.

Bernard, now a young lawyer, is on his way to Washington to argue a case. He'll be staying with friends who have a tennis court. Willy is impressed, and, to counter Bernard's obvious success, tells him that Biff is "doing very big things in the West," but is in town now because Bill Oliver, a sporting goods dealer, has offered him a job.

But for once Willy Loman runs out of words. Nearly breaking down with emotion, he asks Bernard what the secret is that he learned and Biff so clearly missed. After 17, after the Ebbets Field game, Biff never went anywhere. His life fell apart. Does Bernard know why?

> *Bernard:* Willy, do you want to talk candidly?
>
> *Willy:* I regard you as a very brilliant man, Bernard. I value your advice.

We remember that Willy has said those same words to Ben: "I value your advice." Now here he is asking advice from the once-scrawny kid Bernard, whom he scornfully used to call "anemic."

NOTE: Advice is something Willy gives freely to other people, but also needs himself. In spite of his hearty talk, he is not self-confident, and he wonders if he has brought his boys up right. Because his father left when Willy was a baby, he lacked guidance as a young person, and has always felt "temporary" about himself. Contrast Charley, who never gives or asks for advice from anyone.

Bernard does have one idea why Biff never made it. It wasn't flunking math, as Willy thought. Biff was all ready to enroll in summer school. He went up to New England to find Willy and when he got back he was changed. Did Willy have a talk with him?

Willy, so desperate for advice a moment before, now seems full of resentment. Yes, Biff had come to Boston. So what? He obviously remembers something. Bernard continues. Biff had come back from Boston, had a fist fight with Bernard, and burned up his University of Virginia sneakers, the symbol of his bright future. What happened in Boston? Willy becomes defensive. He feels Bernard is blaming him, even though it was Willy himself who brought it up.

Charley comes into the office, urges Bernard to hurry for the train, and gives him a bottle of bourbon as a going-away present. As he leaves, Bernard tells Willy not to worry, that sometimes things don't work out and "it's better for a man just to walk away." Willy can't. "That's when it's tough," says Bernard.

Willy is astonished to find out from Charley that Bernard is going to argue a case in front of the Supreme Court. "And he didn't even mention it!" Willy muses. Willy wonders how Charley brought up Bernard to be so successful, without even "taking an interest" in him.

NOTE: Charley's answer tells a lot about his character. "My salvation is that I never took any interest in anything." This is one reason Willy does not respect Charley: he's not a passionate man with grand hopes and manly talents. It's true that Charley is going to survive and Willy is not, but Willy has no respect for Charley's personality: a man who wears silly-looking knickers his wife bought him, who doesn't care what he eats, and who is content to run a small business. Ironically, Charley has achieved everything Willy wants: financial independence, a distinguished son, two grandsons. These achievements madden Willy, and further emphasize his own wrongheadedness.

After Bernard has left, Charley lays $50 on the desk for Willy. He has been giving him $50 a week ever since Willy went on straight commission. With difficulty Willy asks for $110 to pay his insurance. Charley can't understand why Willy will beg from him, so to speak, but won't accept a job from him. Several times he's offered Willy a position—with no traveling—at $50 a week. But Willy insists he has a job, though at the moment that's a lie.

"What kind of a job is a job without pay?" asks Charley, but Willy is unmovable. "When the hell are you going to grow up?" continues Charley. That's the thing that makes Willy the angriest—remember Charley said the same thing 14 years earlier, just before the Ebbets Field game?—and Willy's literally mad enough to fight. Of course, Charley isn't interested in fighting. Instead in a kind voice he asks his friend how much money he needs.

This is enough to break Willy's proud reserve, and he confesses that he's been fired—by the baby he named Howard in his father's arms. So what? asks Charley. You can't sell sentimental connections. They don't mean anything. Willy has never wanted to believe this. He has preferred to think that if he was "impressive, and well liked" that success would come naturally.

"Why must everyone like you? Who liked J. P. Morgan?" asks Charley. Still, Willy can't accept a job from him, and Charley, angry at his friend's stubbornness, observes that Willy's been jealous of him all along. After he hands him the extra money, Willy muses that after all the traveling, "the appointments, and the years, you end up worth more dead than alive." He's referring to the only thing he has left, his life insurance policy. He doesn't seem to hear Charley when he says, "Willy, nobody's worth nothin' dead." His parting words are a revelation that Willy is beginning to see some truth: "Charley, you're the only friend I got. Isn't that a remarkable thing?" The lights black out.

The new scene, introduced by loud music, is the restaurant where the boys have arranged to treat their father to dinner. Lights come up on Stanley, a waiter who positions a table for Happy, the first to arrive. Evidently a regular customer, Happy orders a special lobster dish made with champagne because the meal is a special occasion to celebrate the business he and Biff plan to start with Bill Oliver's money.

Suddenly Happy notices an attractive woman (his slang for available women is "strudel," meaning a dessert). He tells Stanley to watch while he gets her to go out with him. The line he uses with her is that he's a champagne salesman and he'd like her to try his brand. Notice the ease with which he spins lies to impress her, a "gift of gab" inherited from his father. He is flirting with her when Biff comes in.

Biff is in an emotional turmoil and is not in the mood to flirt with girls. He wants to know if their father has arrived yet, but Happy is too busy playing his game of conquest to answer. Happy tells her that he went to West Point and Biff is a pro football star. Hap offers the girl to Biff as if he owns her. When Biff says he could never impress such a girl, Happy asks where his old confidence is.

NOTE: Like his father, Happy idealizes the golden years of adolescence and promise, when Biff seemed a hero with the world at his feet. It makes Happy uncomfortable to see Biff depressed. If the truth isn't pleasant, Happy, like Willy, varnishes and paints it until it satisfies him. Escaping from uncomfortable truths and putting on an impressive act are his specialties. Now, in the restaurant, Happy can't resist practicing his art, as we will see.

Determined to shake Biff out of what seems to be his nervousness, Happy asks the girl to join them for the evening, and to find a friend. She goes to make a phone call to arrange it. But after she leaves the table Biff quickly tells his brother to cut out the nonsense and listen to what has happened to him. "It's been the strangest day I ever went through."

Biff had waited all day to see his former employer, Mr. Oliver, sending his name in with no success. Naturally Biff by then was beside himself with frustration. At five o'clock Oliver walked out of his office and went home: ". . . he gave me one look and—I realized what a ridiculous lie my whole life has been!" Biff's realization was that he and his family have chosen to believe that instead of a shipping clerk he was a salesman for Oliver.

NOTE: Even Biff himself was convinced of this revised version of events. Exaggeration or revision of past events is a habit with the Lomans. Because they manage to see the past in such glorious terms, they have high expectations of the future. Biff has decided that he must tell his father tonight that he's not the hero Willy's always claimed he was. He wants to end the cycle of revisionism and exaggeration that continually sets standards too high for him to meet. Watch for the dramatic tension of this scene in the restaurant, as Biff's need for truth and Willy's need for fantasy collide.

When Oliver left his office, Biff was full of anger and humiliation at everyone, including himself. "I could've torn the walls down!" he says to Happy, but instead he went into the office and stole Oliver's expensive fountain pen, and ran eleven flights down to the street. Now he's decided to tell this to Willy. No, says Hap, tell him something nice even if you have to make it up: string the story along and it will gradually fade away until Willy's forgotten about it. However, Biff knows perfectly well that Willy never forgets, and, if he tells a lie, "it'll go on forever." Happy is quite right when he says, "Dad is never so happy as when he's looking forward to something!"

NOTE: When Willy's looking forward to something he is counting on it happening his way. When his hopes involve his son's future, this puts unbearable pressure on Biff. Biff feels he's worthless, and that Willy is worthless, too. For years every time he has come home he has felt Willy "mocked" him because he wasn't the prince he was supposed to be. In return, Biff sneered at Willy's efforts to pretend that everything is rosy and glamorous. Willy calls this negative attitude "spite." To spite someone is to treat him or her maliciously for no reason. Is Biff "spiting" Willy? Does Biff have a reason to have turned against his father? Keep these questions in mind in the next few scenes.

Willy arrives at the restaurant. Biff orders double Scotches all around, and admits to having had a few already. How did it go with Oliver, Willy asks Biff. They're both smiling—Willy encouragingly, Biff reassuringly because he has bad news. Slowly Biff starts to tell about his experience. "Terrific, Pop," Happy interjects, trying to tilt the balance from negative to positive. But Biff persists that as he waited for Oliver he realized some "facts" about his life. Unable to refrain from blaming Willy, he says,

Biff: Who was it, Pop? Who ever said I was a salesman with Oliver?
Willy: Well, you were.
Biff: No, Dad, I was a shipping clerk.
Willy: But you were practically—

NOTE: It's a habit in the Loman family to say "practically" this or "almost" that. It's the way they've rewritten the past. This is what Biff is now rejecting as he tries to make a clean start on the basis of who he is instead of who Willy wants him to be. Listen for the key repetitions of "practically" and "almost."

But when Biff begs his father to "hold on to the facts tonight," Willy interrupts. Does Biff want to lay facts on the line? Okay, here's a fact for the boys to digest: he has been fired. Now what good news do they have that he can take home to Linda?

The boys are utterly shocked. Even the disrespect for him that has become habitual lately has not prepared them for this complete shattering of their image of their father. They try to get more information, but he silences them with, "I'm out!"

NOTE: The stage directions say that he's "driving" his point, which is ironic because "driving" a car is how he lives—and dies. The directions then say Biff is "driven," or pushed, into making up a story to satisfy Willy's terrible demand. The playwright's choice of two forms, active and passive, of the same verb emphasizes the direct effect of Willy's life and dreams on Biff. Incidentally, consider the other uses of the verb "to drive": drive a nail, drive a home run, drive someone into a corner, drive someone crazy, etc.

Biff is being railroaded into a version of his meeting with Oliver that will please the others. In a way the salvation of the family depends on Biff's possibilities in life. But despite their attempts to alter his story, Biff is trying to stick to the facts.

Willy: Very hard man to see, y'know.
Happy: Oh, I know.
Willy: Is that where you had the drinks?
Biff: Yeah, he gave me a couple of—no, no!

He can't go through with the lie. Willy accuses him of not having seen Oliver at all, or of insulting him, and, at a loss how to explain it to Willy's satisfaction, Biff tells him just to "let me out of it" and leave him alone. They are shouting at each other.

Willy: Tell me what happened!
Biff: *(to Happy)* I can't talk to him!

Other voices start to crowd into Willy's head, as they do when he gets upset. Young Bernard is announcing that Biff flunked math. Willy shouts frantically, "Math, math, math!" frightening the boys in the restaurant who do not see the people Willy's imagination has summoned. Spurred by his father's apparent agitation, Biff tries to take hold of the situation by once and for all stating the truth. But at this important moment Willy is far away. He returns to the present just as Biff finishes his story about stealing Oliver's pen. Willy missed the whole thing.

The voices grow more insistent in Willy's head. A hotel operator is paging him. "I'm not in my room!" Willy shouts, to Biff and Hap's confusion. "I'll make good," Biff promises rashly, trying to hold Willy down as he rises in his seat. "No, no, no!" Willy keeps shouting.

By this time Biff feels that his father is out of his mind and the only thing that will calm him is a big lie about Oliver. He is right. Oliver liked the Florida idea and wants to have lunch with me tomorrow, Biff tells him. The effect is amazing: Willy listens, brightens, and then exults, "You got it! You got it!"

Startled by the instantaneous change and the new expectations this lie commits him to, Biff wavers between sticking to it and backing down. "I'm just telling you this so you'll know that I can still make an impression, Pop. And I'll make good somewhere, but I can't go tomorrow, see?" He adds that he wouldn't be able to explain taking the pen, especially since he had been suspected while he worked for Oliver of taking a carton of basketballs. Willy is thrown back into dejection by Biff's backing down, and hurls his worst insult at him:

Willy: Don't you want to be anything?
Biff: Pop, how can I go back?

The argument rages back and forth, Biff claiming he went to see Oliver in the first place because of Willy, and Willy insisting he go back and meet Oliver for lunch the next day. Finally Biff uses the only words that Willy can understand: "I've got no appointment!" And Willy retreats to the only thing he's sure of: "Are you spiting me?"

Willy is especially enraged by Biff because a parallel scene involving Biff is going on in his head at the same time. He is remembering a time in his hotel room when he was lying in bed with The Woman in Boston and someone—Biff—was knocking on the door.

In the midst of Willy's emotional chaos, Miss Forsythe, the girl Happy has asked to arrange a date, arrives at their table with her friend Letta. Introductions are made, and Willy is about to sit down and drink with them all when the voice of The Woman pulls him back to the past. Unable to cope with the realities of the past and the present at the same time, Willy escapes to the washroom.

Biff tells the girls they've just seen a "fine troubled prince." Happy, though, is able to drop all his worries and focus on having a good time. He tries to organize the group for a night on the town. Horrified at Happy's thoughtlessness, Biff accuses his brother—rightly, perhaps—of not giving a damn about their father. Biff pulls out of his pocket the rubber hose he has taken from the cellar, tangible evidence that their father is thinking of killing himself. Biff is terribly upset, and reasons that only Happy, who doesn't care about their father, can help Willy: ". . . help him . . . Help me, help me, I can't bear to look at his face!" Totally undone, Biff runs from the restaurant. The girls are confused, but interested. As the three of them rush out after Biff, one of the girls asks, doesn't Hap want to tell his father where he's going? In a final act of callousness, Happy says, as he leaves the restaurant, "No, that's not my father. He's just a guy."

The scene from the past takes over, accompanied by "raw, sensuous music." Someone is knocking on the door of Willy and The Woman's room. It's a mistake, insists Willy, terrified; someone has the wrong door. But fearing the worst, he pushes The Woman into the bathroom, cautioning her three times not to come out.

Young Biff is at the door. He has come to Boston to ask his father to talk the math teacher into raising his grade from 61 to a passing 65 so he can graduate. Biff has confidence that his father's powers of persuasion can turn any disaster into success. Sure, says Willy, I'll go home with you right now. Biff is relieved, and confesses that the math teacher hates him because he overheard Biff make fun of his lisp to entertain the class. Father and son laugh at the joke, but before Willy can hustle Biff out of the room, The Woman joins the laughter and comes out of the bathroom in her slip. Naturally Biff is horrified. Though Willy makes excuses—there's a party in her room, her room is being painted—Biff realizes that his father is having an affair. He is deeply shocked.

Though he is trying to push her out the door in her underwear, the offended woman won't go until Willy gives her the stockings he promised her. This is the final outrage for Biff, who senses how intimate a gift this is. Assuming a brisk manner after the woman has gone, Willy tries to gloss over the crisis, alternately pleading and ordering Biff not to cry. But all the boy's determination and trust are gone. The teacher won't listen to you, Biff says, and I'm not going to college.

NOTE: More upsetting even than Biff's disappointment about his own plans is his disillusionment about his father's character. He has surely known all along that Willy exaggerates, but he never suspected that his fabrications covered ignoble deeds like this one. Biff has always been carried along on the crest of his father's fantasies, and now as his image of Willy comes crashing down, his image of himself is shattered, too.

Willy is stern with Biff, but Biff is inconsolable. His weeping pierces Willy to the heart. Willy explains that the woman means nothing to him, he was just lonely, but Biff's reply shows that he sees only Willy's betrayal: "You gave her Mama's stockings!"

NOTE: Stockings are a symbol in this play. Thrifty people mended their stockings with special silk thread. It was Linda's mending her stockings that brought back the memory to Willy of the woman in the hotel. He can't stand to see Linda mending stockings because it makes him feel guilty about his affair.

When sixteen-year-old Biff recovers from crying, only anger and scorn are left for his father. Calling him a liar, fake, and phony, he leaves with his suitcase. Willy, who has knelt down to comfort Biff, is left on his knees, and that is where we see him when the lights and music bring us back to the restaurant.

Stanley helps Willy to his feet and brushes him off. He slips the tip Willy has given him back into Willy's coat, explaining that Happy has already paid him. Willy hurries out. Suddenly he feels the need to buy some seeds and plant a garden.

We hear the flute as the lights come up on the kitchen. The boys have arrived home with roses to try to pacify the anger they know their mother will have for them. She knocks the roses to the floor and tells them exactly what she thinks of them: that they don't care if their father lives or dies, that there's no stranger they would desert in such a time of trouble, and that they are to get out and not come back.

Happy simply denies all the accusations, lying blatantly that Willy "had a swell time with us." But Linda isn't even looking at him. As usual, Biff is the center of attention and Happy is on the periphery. When Linda orders him to pick the flowers up off the floor—"I'm not your maid any more"—Happy refuses and goes upstairs.

Stooping to pick up the flowers, Biff admits everything: "Now you hit it on the nose! The scum of the earth, and you're looking at him!" He may have acted like a "louse," he persists, but before he gets out of the house he has to talk to Willy. Against Linda's wishes, he goes outside to find his father.

Willy is planting seeds by flashlight and having a conversation with Ben who, as we know, appears when Willy needs advice. They are discussing a business deal that will make $20,000 for Biff. It is, of course, Willy's notion of killing himself to cash in on his life insurance policy: the final sale of his last resource, his own life.

NOTE: Willy seems eager and optimistic about the proposition. The prospect of setting Biff up financially has far more meaning to him than continuing to live a life that he now sees will never be what he dreamed of for himself. He is now completely transferring that dream onto his son. Unfortunately, it's the very dream Biff resents and rejects. The idea of making $20,000 appeals to Willy because it's the kind of deal he's always longed to swing. It's not an "appointment," that intangible, uncertain arrangement he's been dependent on all his life. This is "guaranteed, gilt-edged," a concrete profit he can see "like a diamond, shining in the dark."

Ben, speaking for Willy's subconscious mind, raises possible objections: the insurance inspectors might not honor the policy; it might be called cowardly; Biff might hate you and call you a damned fool. Willy can refute all but the last, and because he's doing this for Biff, he can't stand the idea of Biff hating him. How can we get back to the wonderful past, he laments, when we always had something good to look forward to?

Biff intrudes on Willy's conversation and brings him back to the present. He wants to say goodbye and leave on good terms. They argue again about Oliver. Biff realizes he can't talk to his father rationally, and finally just says it would be best if he left no forwarding address. Going into the house, Willy refuses to shake Biff's hand, and then prevents him from going by saying,

> *Willy:* May you rot in hell if you leave this house!
> *Biff:* Exactly what is it that you want from me?

Willy is moved almost to poetry by the intensity of his emotion: "Spite, spite, is the word of your undoing!" Biff answers, and we feel that at last it is the truth: "I'm not blaming it on you!" but Willy isn't listening, nothing seems to make him hear what Biff is saying. So Biff does the thing everyone dreads most: he is direct and confronts Willy with the rubber tube, evidence of Willy's intention to commit suicide. This will not make a hero of you, warns Biff. Now let's lay it on the line: "We never told the truth for ten minutes in this house!" Biff starts listing the big lies: Happy is not the assistant buyer but a lowly assistant to the assistant. He himself had no address because he was in jail for stealing:

> *Biff:* I stole myself out of every good job since high school!
> *Willy:* And whose fault is that?
> *Biff:* And I never got anywhere because you blew me so full of hot air I could never stand taking orders from anybody! That's whose fault it is!

This is the moment of truth for Biff, and for the family. "I'm through with it!" he says. He's going to stop stealing, admit that he's not "a leader of men," and start over. During this scene he has begun to call his father by his first name, Willy, as man to man, rather than Pop. But Willy rejects it all with "You vengeful, spiteful mut!"

Seeing that all his words mean nothing, Biff grabs his father as if to shake sense into him. He is furious. "Pop, I'm nothing! I'm nothing, Pop. Can't you understand that? There's no spite in it any more. I'm just what I am, that's all." He breaks into sobs. Willy holds his face. He's astonished and moved to see Biff clinging to him and crying. Exhausted and empty, Biff pulls away and goes upstairs, saying he'll leave in the morning.

Willy's mood has changed completely. From raging anger to defensiveness, he has come to gentle wonderment. To Linda and Happy he says, "Isn't that—isn't that remarkable? Biff—he likes me!" He loves you, he always has, Linda and Hap assure him.

Willy is ecstatic. "He cried! Cried to me. That boy—that boy is going to be magnificent!" Has Willy learned anything from Biff? Has he listened to the truthful, hurtful things Biff has been saying to them all? No. Here he is, dreaming his same old dream again.

Full of the feeling of promise for the future, of forgiveness for the past, Willy can hardly wait to rush out and do what he has to do. When Linda, urging him to come to bed, says, "It's all settled now," the words have different meanings to the two of them: for her it means Biff will leave and you won't fight anymore; for Willy it means Biff loves me and the only thing I have left to give him is $20,000.

On his way upstairs Happy chimes in with his customary attention-getting line: he's going to get married and be head of his department before the year is up. As usual, no one pays any notice to him.

Ben is on the scene again, on the edge of the shadows. He is not a remembered figure now, but a personification of Willy's own feelings. "The jungle is dark but full of diamonds, Willy," says Ben. This means Willy is frightened of what he has to do, but the reward is worth it.

Sending Linda to bed, saying he just wants to sit alone for a few minutes, Willy imagines what Biff will be like with a fortune of $20,000 behind him. When the insurance check comes "he'll be ahead of Bernard again!" The old competitive drive races in him, the only credo Willy has ever lived by.

As Ben drifts away, Willy is wrapped up in a moment fifteen years before when he was giving advice to Biff on how to win the football game. Suddenly realizing he's alone, Willy is now the one who needs advice. "Ben, where do I . . . ? Ben, how do I . . . ?" Hearing Linda calling him, hearing the high, screaming music, Willy rushes offstage and we hear the car roaring off.

Though we don't hear the actual car crash, the music crashes and then dies, becoming one sad note as Linda, Biff, Happy, Charley, and Bernard slowly gather. As they put on their coats, the music becomes a funeral march, the light changes from night to day. They come forward, and Linda lays down a bunch of flowers on a spot that is Willy's grave.

REQUIEM

As dark falls in the cemetery, Linda stares at the grave. She is wondering why nobody came to the funeral. (She is thinking of the hundreds of people who reportedly turned up for the funeral of Dave Singleman, Willy's hero.) She can't understand why Willy died now, just when all their bills are paid. "He only needed a little salary," she says, but Charley answers wisely, "No man only needs a little salary."

NOTE: What did Willy need? He needed love, respect, and triumph. He needed glamor and success and to be thought of as impressive.

Everyone in the play has a different verdict on Willy. "He had the wrong dreams," says Biff. "A salesman is got to dream, boy. It comes with the territory," replies Charley. Hap adds, "It's the only dream you can have—to come out number-one man."

Is it? They all acknowledge "there's more of him in that front stoop than in all the sales he ever made." "He never knew who he was," claims Biff. But Happy, heir to the same dreams as his father, is determined to see that his father didn't die in vain. "I'm staying right in this city, and I'm gonna beat this racket! . . . He fought it out here, and this is where I'm gonna win it for him." Biff just shakes his head and says, "I know who I am."

Linda is heartbroken and bewildered. She doesn't understand why Willy killed himself. To the end she was in love with both sides of this paradoxical man: his dream and the suffering of his failures. She has worked to keep the family afloat with what little money he brought home, and finally they are paid up. "I can't understand it, Willy. I made the last payment on the house today. Today, dear. And there'll be nobody home. We're free and clear. We're free. . . We're free . . . "

NOTE: The family are also free, finally, of Willy's dreams. How will this affect them now? His expectations are ingrained in their lives. They are free to find out who they are. When Biff says "I know who I am" he means, I'm nobody but myself. If Happy said the same thing, he would mean, I'm somebody. Linda is free to grow old and die, no longer having to care for her husband who never grew up. The house is free to begin to decay, lacking Willy's handyman skills. All are free to live and die, as all things must, leaving nothing behind them. Only the music of the flute plays on, while "the hard towers of the apartment buildings rise into sharp focus."

A STEP BEYOND

Tests and Answers

TESTS

Test 1

1. The opening references to Willy Loman's driving ability _____
   A. serve as introduction to his growing senility
   B. set us up for the action at the end of the play
   C. are signs that Willy's family doesn't care about him

2. The tantalizing thing about brother Ben's success in the African jungle is _____
   A. its seeming lack of effort
   B. that Willy cannot appreciate it
   C. that Willy is unable to share in Ben's good fortune

3. "A man is not a bird, to come and go with the springtime" is spoken by Linda to _____
   A. Biff
   B. Willy
   C. Hap

4. In her famous speech ("Attention must be paid"), Linda Loman is scolding _____
   A. Willy's insensitive employer
   B. her sons, Biff and Happy
   C. Uncle Charley

5. Linda is upset over ______
   I. the length of rubber pipe behind the heater
   II. Willy's probable suicide attempts
   III. Willy's extramarital affairs
   A. I and II only
   B. I and III only
   C. II and III only

6. Willy uses the death of a salesman story to make a point to ______
   A. Biff and Happy
   B. young Bernard, his neighbor's son
   C. his boss, Howard

7. Arthur Miller's often quoted words which have become a common expression are ______
   I. "You can't eat the orange and throw the peel away"
   II. "He's . . . riding on a smile and a shoeshine"
   III. "It's who you know and the smile on your face"
   A. I and II only
   B. I and III only
   C. I, II, and III

8. Biff's failure to graduate from high school was related to ______
   A. his arrogance about study
   B. his obsession with sports
   C. his visit to his father in Boston

9. Out of frustration following his "non-interview" with Bill Oliver, Biff ______
   A. maliciously pulled the fire alarm in his office
   B. stole the man's fountain pen

C. smashed the window in the showroom

10. The immaturity of Biff and Happy is seen ______
    I. when they leave Willy alone in the restaurant
    II. in their plans for a sporting goods partnership
    III. in their appeal for help to Uncle Charley
  A. I and II only
  B. II and III only
  C. I, II, and III

11. A basic theme of *Death of a Salesman* is the distortion of the "American dream." What is Willy's relation to this?

12. What is the unique form Arthur Miller devised for *Death of a Salesman*, and how does it work?

13. Describe the contradictions Willy's character, and give examples.

14. Discuss the use of symbols in the play.

15. Arthur Miller is a skillful writer for the theater. Analyze his language in *Death of a Salesman*.

Test 2

1. Biff refers to himself as a "bum" ______
  A. and his father agrees tearfully
  B. but his father still thinks of him as "magnificent"
  C. and Willy says, "You're a bum in spades!"

2. Happy could best be described as ______
  A. upwardly mobile
  B. hedonistic
  C. family oriented

3. Linda called her sons ____
   I. "the scum of the earth"
   II. "you pseudo-intellectuals"
   III. "a pair of animals"
   A. I and II only
   B. I and III only
   C. II and III only

4. In Willy's mind the insurance money would go ____
   A. to help Biff become a success
   B. to pay off all of their debts
   C. to repay Linda for all the pain he had caused her

5. In the big showdown near the play's end, Biff protests that ____
   A. none of the Loman men ever told the truth
   B. his father's meddling caused him to fail in business
   C. he never had a fair chance to make it in life

6. One of the ironies attached to Willy's suicide is that ____
   A. the play implies that the insurance company did not honor the policy
   B. their mortgage had finally been paid off
   C. he claimed to be a good driver

7. Willy would have been disappointed with ____
   A. Linda's tribute at the graveside
   B. Biff's plans for spending the $20,000
   C. the poor attendance at his funeral

8. In Charley's requiem for Willy, he said, ____
   A. "A salesman is got to dream, boy. It comes with the territory"

B. "Nobody's worth nothin' dead"
C. "He had his damn priorities all mixed up"

9. When Willy says, "They'll come from Maine, Massachusetts, Vermont, New Hampshire! All the old timers with the strange license plates," he is talking about ______
A. the New England customers for Biff's sporting goods
B. his own funeral
C. his imaginary into the Salesmen's Hall of Fame

10. What has Biff been doing out West? ______
A. setting up a sporting goods store
B. working at seasonal outdoor jobs
C. playing pro football

11. Linda is the only major female character in the play. Discuss her influence on Willy.

12. How do Ben and Charley, both of whom have been "successful," represent opposite extremes for Willy?

13. The relationships between fathers and sons are important in this play. Contrast Willy's relationship with his father, Willy's with Biff and Happy, and Charley's with Bernard.

14. Analyze the degree of self-understanding Willy achieves before he kills himself.

15. Discuss how the Requiem affects our view of the whole play.

ANSWERS

Test 1

1. B 2. A 3. A 4. B 5. A 6. C
7. C 8. C 9. B 10. A

11. Willy believes the Capitalist promise that anyone who tries can make good in business. He feels that if he is "well liked" he will become successful, and he teaches this credo to his sons. When none of them becomes rich or popular, Willy, Biff, and Happy try shortcuts to success by bending the rules of proper business conduct. Then they lie to themselves and each other about how successful they are. (See section on Themes.)

12. Miller combined scenes from Willy's past and present. The scenes are acted on the same stage by the same people, dressed alternately as they are now and as they looked fifteen years earlier. Unlike flashbacks, the scenes from the past are actually happening in Willy's mind in the present. (See section on Point of View and Form.)

13. Willy's paradoxical nature stems from his refusal to admit what his character is, and his insistence on trying to be someone he's not. Therefore, he works as a salesman but can't make any money at it. He will borrow money from Charley, but he won't take a job from him. He is good with his hands, but he won't view that as a measure of success. (See section on The Characters.)

14. *Death of a Salesman* is partly expressionistic. This means that many of the central ideas are conveyed through symbols. (See section on Influences.) Symbols involving nature versus the city are the flute, the leaf pattern cast by the stage lights, and the outlines of the towering apartment buildings. (See Notes on each of these.) Other symbols are the stockings Linda is mending while, unknown to her, Willy is giving new stockings to another woman; the sample cases Willy carries on in the first act and is asked to return when he is fired in Act II; the diamonds Ben found, and Willy's claim in Act II that "a man can end with diamonds here on the basis of being rich," and the comparison of Willy's final "deal"—suicide—to a diamond.

15. Miller blends ordinary and poetic language. (See Language section.) He manages to reproduce a natural, colloquial American speech pattern that is colorful and memorable. The different characters and the poignancy of their situations are conveyed through the dialogue.

Test 2

1. B **2.** B **3.** B **4.** A **5.** A **6.** B
7. C **8.** A **9.** B **10.** B

11. Linda is Willy's comfort and support. (See The Characters section.) She believes in him completely, even in his fantasy of himself. When Ben comes and offers Willy a faraway job, she boycotts it, saying he ought to be satisfied with his wonderful position at home. Willy needed her unconditional approval, but ironically it may have blocked the one chance he had to escape to a more suitable way of life.

12. Willy reveres Ben and scorns Charley. He has made Ben into a symbol of success. (See section on The Characters.) Because of his ambitions and dapper personality, Ben somehow ended up with diamond mines. When Willy feels discouraged, he consults his imaginary picture of Ben. On the other hand, Charley is a man without grand ambitions, for himself or his son. Willy has no respect for Charley's inability with tools, his ignorance of sports, and his general lack of passion.

13. Willy never knew his father well, and feels the resulting lack of guidance all his life. Because he himself longs for advice, Willy is constantly giving advice to his sons, especially Biff, his favorite. Biff strives to meet his father's expectations until he catches his father with another woman. Disillusioned, Biff rejects everything about Willy, particularly his "phony dream," as he calls it in their final fight. Biff and Willy's relationship ultimately becomes a power struggle, which leaves Happy in the shadows. Happy fails to get attention from his father, ending up with the same kinds of insecurities and compensating illusions as Willy. Charley takes no interest in his son Bernard, nor in anything, he claims, which mystifies Willy because Bernard turns into a successful lawyer and father. (See The Characters section on Bernard.)

14. Critics have said that a tragic hero must discover or recognize something important about himself before he dies. (See Themes section.) Although Willy is not an intellectual, the play chronicles his growing self-awareness. The author feels that the play can be seen as Willy's "confession." Miller points out that Willy realizes that his life has been lived in vain, or he would never have been moved to commit suicide. Ben suggests suicide might be cowardly, but Willy's answer is honest: "Does it take more guts to stand here the rest of my life ringing up a zero?" Even in his hour of death, Willy's clearest images are drawn from the world of selling.

15. The short Requiem gives all the major characters a chance to pronounce their judgments on Willy. We learn here what the people who cared about him really feel about his "dream" of himself. These are important clues as to how they will go on now that they are "free" of Willy's expectations. (See final Note.) He led a courageous but futile life, and in that respect he resembles many of us.

Term Paper Ideas

1. How do Miller's own life experiences enter into the play?

2. What was Miller's social objective in writing this play?

3. Do you admire Charley and Bernard? Why or why not?

4. Discuss Willy's skill at revising incidents: list actual incidents and what he turns them into.

5. List and discuss the ways men compete in this play: sports, money, women, possessions, success of their children.

6. Write a character analysis of Willy, discussing his strengths and weaknesses.

7. Do Linda and Willy have a good marriage?

8. Why does Biff say he's "mixed up"? How much of it is his father's fault?

9. Contrast the characters of Biff and Happy. Would they make a good team?

10. Which character or characters most engage your sympathy? Why?

11. Contrast Willy's and Charley's personalities. Which would you rather have as a neighbor?

12. Discuss the women in the play from the point of view of women's liberation.

13. Should Willy have been a builder (carpenter)?

14. List and discuss the aspects of Miller's language that make the play so moving.

15. Is Willy a good father?

16. Should Howard Wagner have found (or created) a job for Willy in New York?

17. Discuss the importance of music in the play.

18. Trace references to trees and plants and growing.

19. What different things do Willy and Biff learn about themselves?

20. Discuss the elements of Happy's nature that come from each of his parents.

21. Why is the character of Ben in the play?

22. What is the function of the Requiem?

23. Analyze the play as though its title were *The Inside of His Head*.

24. What does Willy have to remember? Why now?

25. Discuss the form of the play as a reflection of Willy's state of mind.

26. Discuss why Willy commits suicide and what he feels he achieves by it.

27. Describe the relative influences of Greek tragedy and German expressionism on the form of the play.

28. Is Willy a "little man"?

29. List actors you would like to see play Willy, and what qualities in him each actor would bring out.

30. Analyze transitions from present to past and back to present.

31. Do you see Willy as a tragic figure?

Further Reading

CRITICAL WORKS

Death of a Salesman has frequently been written about. In the list below are two collections of essays about this play alone. All of the books should be readily available in school and community libraries.

Bentley, Eric. *In Search of Theatre*. New York: Knopf, 1953, pp. 84–87. Bentley, a controversial critic and theorist, stands out among the writers critical of the play.

Clurman, Harold, ed. *The Portable Arthur Miller*. New York: Viking, 1971. Clurman, a noted director and an exceptional critic, knew Arthur Miller well and directed several of his plays. The Biographical Notes and Editor's Introduction are, therefore, a particularly sound source.

Corrigan, Robert W., ed. *Arthur Miller: A Collection of Critical Essays*. Englewood Cliffs, N.J.: Prentice-Hall, 1969. Ten essays give a picture of the whole of Miller's theater work to the date of publication. This book is one source for Brian Parker's "Point of View in Arthur Miller's *Death of a Salesman*."

Gassner, John. "*Death of a Salesman:* First Impressions, 1949," in *The Theatre in Our Times*. New York: Crown, 1954, pp. 364–73. One of the most distinguished American critics includes in this book two reviews of *Death of a Salesman*, one published just after the production opened on Broadway and the second six months later.

Hogan, Robert. *Arthur Miller*. Minneapolis: University of Minnesota Press, 1964, Pamphlets on American Writers, No. 40. A thoughtful, easy-to-read 45 pages that give a biographical background and discuss all of Miller's work through *After the Fall*.

Kazan, Elia. "Excerpts from the notebook kept in preparation for directing *Death of a Salesman*," Kenneth Thorpe Rowe, in *A Theater in Your Head*. New York: Funk & Wagnalls, 1960, pp. 44–59. These notes by the brilliant director of the original production are an exciting glimpse of the play before it became a classic.

Koon, Helene Wickham, ed. *Twentieth Century Interpretations of* Death of a Salesman: *A Collection of Critical Essays.* Englewood Cliffs, N.J.: Prentice-Hall, 1983. Eleven appreciative essays on every aspect of the play. Koon's "Introduction," Brian Parker's "Point of View in Arthur Miller's *Death of a Salesman,*" and Lois Gordon's "*Death of a Salesman*: An Appreciation" are the most helpful.

Krutch, Joseph Wood. *The American Drama Since 1918*, rev. ed. New York: Random House, 1957, pp. 325–329. A literate and humanistic American critic considers Miller and *Death of a Salesman* in relation to the other new plays of the time, Tennessee Williams' *A Streetcar Named Desire* and the last plays of Eugene O'Neill.

Miller, Arthur, *The Theater Essays of Arthur Miller*, ed. Robert A. Martin. New York: Viking, 1978. Miller has written extensively about the theater and his work. He is always stimulating and sometimes contradictory. Of special importance for *Death of a Salesman* are "Tragedy and the Common Man," "The *Salesman* Has a Birthday," "Introduction to the *Collected Plays,*" and "Arthur Miller: An Interview."

Moss, Leonard. *Arthur Miller*, rev. ed. Boston: Twayne Publishers, 1980. An exhaustive examination of Miller's work and themes, play by play, the book also includes a lengthy "Conversation with Arthur Miller."

Tynan, Kenneth, "American Blues: The Plays of Arthur Miller and Tennessee Williams," in *Curtains*, New York: Atheneum, 1961, pp. 257–66. An outstanding British critic views the work of the two American playwrights, with several perceptive paragraphs on *Death of a Salesman.*

Weales, Gerald, ed. *Arthur Miller: Death of a Salesman, Text and Criticism*. New York: Viking, 1967. A rich resource book, this volume contains the text of the play and all of

Miller's related essays, as well as an instructive article by Jo Mielziner, the designer of the original production, about how his ideas contributed to the final form of the play. Harold Clurman's review of the first Broadway production, "The Success Dream on the American Stage," is here, as well as psychoanalyst Daniel E. Schneider's article "Play of Dreams," an excerpt from his book, *The Psychoanalyst and the Artist.* Articles critical of *Death of a Salesman* include those by Eleanor Clark and John Gassner.

Welland, Dennis. *Arthur Miller.* New York: Grove Press, 1961. A balanced and scholarly review of Miller's work, both plays and fiction, through *A View from the Bridge.* The chapter on *Death of a Salesman* fairly summarizes criticism of the play and answers the major arguments.

AUTHOR'S OTHER WORKS

Situation Normal (reportage), 1944
The Man Who Had All the Luck (play), *1944*
Focus (novel), 1945
All My Sons (play), 1947
An Enemy of the People (adaptation of Henrik Ibsen's play), 1951
The Crucible (play), 1953
A Memory of Two Mondays (one-act play), 1955
A View from the Bridge (one-act play), 1955
A View from the Bridge (full-length version), 1957
Arthur Miller's Collected Plays, 1957
The Misfits (screenplay), 1961
Jane's Blanket (children's story), 1963
After the Fall (play), 1964
Incident at Vichy (play), 1965
I Don't Need You Any More (short stories), 1967
The Price (play), 1968

In Russia (reportage), 1969
The Creation of the World and Other Business (play), 1973
In the Country (reportage), 1977
The Theater Essays of Arthur Miller, 1978
Chinese Encounters (reportage), 1979
Playing for Time (television play), 1980
The American Clock (play), 1980
Two by A.M. (one-act plays), 1983
Salesman in Beijing (reportage), 1984

The Critics

. . . My father is, literally, a much more realistic guy than Willy Loman, and much more successful as a personality. And he'd be the last man in the world to ever commit suicide. Willy is based on an individual whom I knew very little, who was a salesman; it was years later that I realized I had only seen that man about a total of four hours in twenty years. He gave one of those impressions that is basic, evidently. When I thought of him, he would simply be a mute man: he said no more than two hundred words to me. I was a kid. Later on, I had another of that kind of contact, with a man whose fantasy was always overreaching his real outline. I've always been aware of that kind of an agony, of someone who has some driving, implacable wish in him which never goes away, which he can never block out. And it broods over him, it makes him happy sometimes or it makes him suicidal, but it never leaves him. Any hero whom we even begin to think of as tragic is obsessed, whether it's Lear or Hamlet or the women in the Greek plays.—"Arthur Miller: An Interview," *The Paris Review*, Summer 1966

Obviously, *Death of a Salesman* is a criticism of the moral and social standards of contemporary America, not merely a record of the particular plight of one man. And, also obviously, it presents Willy as a victim of the deterioration of the "American dream," the belief in untrammelled individualism. The word "dream" is a key word, recurring frequently in the play; and the deterioration of American individualism is traced through the Loman generations in a descending scale, from the Whitman-like exuberance of Willy's father, through Ben, Willy himself, to the empty predatoriness of Happy, who is he admits, compulsively competitive in sex and business for no reason at all.—Brian Parker, "Point of View in Arthur Miller's *Death of a Salesman*," *University of Toronto Quarterly*, January 1966

So Willy Loman wreaks havoc on his own life and on that of his sons. The blight of his own confusion is visited upon them. Unaware of what warped his mind and behavior, he commits suicide in the conviction that a legacy of twenty thousand dollars is all that is needed to save his beloved but almost equally damaged offspring. This may not be "tragic," but such distorted thinking maims a very great number of folk in the world today.—Harold Clurman, "Editor's Introduction," *The Portable Arthur Miller*, 1971

The particulars concerning Willy's situation also have universal significance. Willy has lived passionately for values to which he is committed, and he comes to find that they are false and inadequate. He has loved his sons with a passion which wanted for them that which would destroy them. He has grown old and he will soon vanish without a trace, and he discovers really the vanity of all human endeavor, save perhaps love. His foolishness is really no greater than Othello's raving jealousy or Lear's appreciation of the insincere, outward appearance of love. A pension would not help him, nor, had he come to be J. P. Morgan would it have helped. Linda says, "A small man can be just as exhausted as a great man," and she cries out "Attention must be paid." Inevitably, no matter what material heights a man succeeds to, his life is brief and his comprehension finite, while the universe remains infinite and incomprehensible. Willy comes to face, if you will, the absurdity of life, and it is for this reason that attention must be paid."—Lois Gordon, "*Death of a Salesman:* An Appreciation," *The Forties: Fiction, Poetry, Drama*, 1969

Willy Loman, exhausted salesman, does not go back to the past. The past, as in hallucination, comes back to him; not chronologically as in flashback, but *dynamically with the inner logic of his erupting volcanic unconscious.* In psychiatry we call this "the return of the repressed," when a mind breaks under the invasion of primitive impulses no longer capable of compromise with reality.—Daniel E. Schneider, M.D., *The Psychoanalyst and the Artist*, 1950

Willy is one vast contradiction, and this contradiction is his downfall. He is a nicer guy than Charley. He is so nice, as someone said once, he's got to end up poor. This makes Charley untroubled and a success, and Willy contradictory, neurotic, full of love and longing, need for admiration and affection, full of a sense of worthlessness and inadequacy and dislocation *and a failure.*—Elia Kazan, "Notebook," in *A Theater in Your Head*, 1960

Sonja LK Dez. 89
S. 87 Nr. 13
S. 29 Aristotle
Requiem